second edition

Clinical Procedures *in*

Therapeutic Exercise

second edition
2

Clinical Procedures *in*
Therapeutic Exercise

Patricia Sullivan, PhD, PT
Associate Professor, Physical Therapy Program
Institute of Health Professions
Massachusetts General Hospital
Boston, Massachusetts
Lecturer, Department of Orthopaedic Surgery
Harvard Medical School
Cambridge, Massachusetts

Prudence Markos, MS, PT
Senior Physical Therapist, Physical Therapy Services
Assistant Professor, Physical Therapy Program
Institute of Health Professions
Massachusetts General Hospital
Boston, Massachusetts

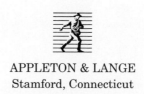

APPLETON & LANGE
Stamford, Connecticut

Notice: The authors and the publisher of this volume have taken care that the
information and recommendations contained herein are accurate and compatible
with the standards generally accepted at the time of publication. Nevertheless,
it is difficult to ensure that all the information given is entirely accurate
for all circumstances. The publisher disclaims any liability, loss, or damage
incurred as a consequence, directly or indirectly, of the use and application
of any of the contents of this volume.

Copyright © 1996 by Appleton & Lange
A Simon & Schuster Company
Copyright © 1987 by Appleton & Lange
A Publishing Division of Prentice-Hall

96 97 98 99 00 / 10 9 8 7 6 5 4 3 2 1

Prentice Hall International (UK) Limited, *London*
Prentice Hall of Australia Pty. Limited, *Sydney*
Prentice Hall Canada, Inc., *Toronto*
Prentice Hall Hispanoamericana, S.A., *Mexico*
Prentice Hall of India Private Limited, *New Delhi*
Prentice Hall of Japan, Inc., *Tokyo*
Simon & Schuster Asia Pte. Ltd., *Singapore*
Editora Prentice Hall do Brasil Ltda., *Rio de Janeiro*
Prentice Hall, *Upper Saddle River, New Jersey*

Sullivan, Patricia E., 1946–
    Clinical procedures in therapeutic exercise / Patricia Sullivan,
Prudence Markos. — 2nd ed.
        p.   cm.
    Includes bibliographical references and index.
    ISBN 0-8385-1339-5 (pbk. : alk. paper)
    1. Exercise therapy.   I. Markos, Prudence D., 1940-
II. Title.
    [DNLM: 1. Exercise Therapy—methods.   WB 541 S951c 1996]
    RM725.S838   1996
    615.8′2—dc20
    DNLM/DLC
    for Library of Congress   95-24975
                                                                  CIP

ISBN 0-8385-1339-5

Acquisitions Editor: Cheryl L. Mehalik
Production Service: Rainbow Graphics, Inc.
Designer: Janice Barsevich Bielawa

PRINTED IN THE UNITED STATES OF AMERICA

Contents

How to Use This Book

The main purpose of this text is to instruct the reader, in a step-by-step manner, how to perform therapeutic exercise procedures. This book may be used as a complement to our text, *Clinical Decision Making in Therapeutic Exercise,* which emphasizes the theory and formulation of therapeutic exercise procedures.

Each exercise procedure is composed of three segments: activity, technique, and parameter. This division provides the therapist with a consistent framework to evaluate and treat patients, and to serve as a guide in the progression of the treatment plan. The three segments are defined as:

- **Activity (A).** The posture and movement patterns occurring in that posture, chosen to achieve the functional outcomes of intervention.
- **Technique (T).** Type of muscle contraction, either concentric, eccentric, or isometric, and the sensory input used to achieve the stages of movement control.
- **Parameter (P).** The frequency, intensity, and duration of movement chosen to enhance movement capacity.

An example of how this would be written in an exercise program is:

- **A**—Supine: hip and knee extension.
- **T**—Shortened held resisted contraction (isometric contractions of gluteals and quadriceps).
- **P**—Maintained at 40% intensity for 10 seconds; as a home exercise performed 2x/day for 10 repetitions each.

In the initial section of this text, patterns of movement (trunk, bilateral, unilateral) are described. We suggest they be performed first as active movement for ease of learning. The next sections describe treatment procedures emphasizing the activities and techniques. The mat procedures are sequenced to promote stages of movement control within each posture. Patient's impairments and the goals of physical therapy are indicated for each procedure along with a detailed description of the exercise application. In addition, the reader is alerted to common problems with application that may be avoided with attention to either body mechanics, placement of manual contacts, or amount and direction of resistive forces. Problem-oriented worksheets are included which guide the reader in the sequencing and application of the previously described procedures to achieve stated goals.

A section on equipment focuses on the use of wall pulleys. In this section, variations of pulley height and angle of pull to optimize resistance are addressed. Adaptation of the pulley program with elastic bands is illustrated for home use.

To assist the therapist in developing a treatment plan, several examples of intervention models for patients with either orthopaedic or neurologic deficits are depicted. The procedures suggested in this section correspond to the numbered procedures in the body of the text for easy referencing.

Readers are encouraged to practice all procedures on subjects without physical impairments to learn the patterns of movement and techniques, and most importantly to develop an appreciation of normal responses. Once this is accomplished, procedures can be applied more skillfully in treatment to meet each patient's needs. In time and with perseverance, a therapist can develop a wide repertoire of skills applicable to all patients.

While this text addresses the use of therapeutic exercise procedures, therapists must remember that other forms of intervention, such as modalities and joint mobilization, may need to be incorporated into the total treatment plan.

Acknowledgments

We are grateful for the support and confidence afforded us by our families, friends, and colleagues. The authors would like to thank the following people for their assistance in the development of this text: Mary Alice Minor, Simon Adey, Mike Roberson, Leslie Butterfield-Boyd, Maryann Conway, and Nancy DeMuth. We thank the students in the Therapeutic Exercise course at Massachusetts General Institute of Health Professions, and at Boston University. In addition, we thank the Physical Therapy Department, Massachusetts General Hospital, for the use of their department during photographic sessions. Photographs were taken by Lucia Littlefield and Patricia Sullivan.

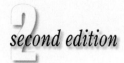

second edition

Clinical Procedures *in*

Therapeutic Exercise

part one

Patterns

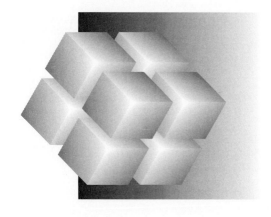

Patterns of Movement

Chapter Outline

Key Terms

Active Movement (**AM**)
Bilateral Asymmetrical (**BA**)
Bilateral Reciprocal (**BR**)
Bilateral Symmetrical (**BS**)
Combining Components
Cross Diagonal (**CD**)
Diagonal 1 Extension (**D1E**)
Diagonal 2 Extension (**D2E**)
Diagonal 1 Flexion (**D1F**)
Diagonal 2 Flexion (**D2F**)
Head and Trunk Motion
Prime Movers
Reciprocal Asymmetrical
Reversing Movements
Rolling
Static–Dynamic
Trunk Movement
Unidirectional Movement
Upper Trunk Extension (Lift)
Upper Trunk Flexion (Chop)

DEFINITIONS

D2 Flexion (D2F)

Combining Components: scapular elevation, adduction and upward rotation • shoulder flexion, abduction, external rotation • forearm supination • wrist, finger, and thumb radial extension

Prime Movers—scapula and shoulder—trapezius • middle deltoid

D2 Extension (D2E)

Combining Components: scapular depression, abduction, and downward rotation • shoulder extension, adduction and internal rotation • forearm pronation • wrist and finger ulnar flexion • thumb opposition

Prime Movers—scapula and shoulder—pectoralis minor • sternal portion of the pectoralis major

D1 Flexion (D1F)

Combining Components: scapular elevation, abduction, upward rotation • shoulder flexion, adduction, external rotation • forearm supination • wrist and finger flexion • thumb adduction

Prime Movers—scapula and shoulder—serratus anterior • anterior deltoid

D1 Extension (D1E)

Combining Components: scapular depression, adduction, downward rotation • shoulder extension, abduction, internal rotation • forearm pronation • wrist and finger ulnar extension • thumb abduction

Prime Movers—scapula and shoulder—rhomboids • middle trapezius • posterior deltoid

Patterns Performed as Active Movements

The upper extremity (UE), lower extremity (LE), and upper trunk diagonal patterns will first be performed actively while standing to learn the movements. These patterns combine movements in the three planes of motion (coronal, sagittal, and transverse) and simulate functional motions.

The term **combining components** is used to describe the simultaneous movement that occurs at each segment within a limb. **Prime movers** are muscles that are responsible for each segmental movement.

1

Activity: Standing; upper extremity (UE) bilateral symmetrical D2 (BSD2)

Technique: Active movement

The activity begins with the arms crossed in D2E (Fig. 1A). The shoulders are extended, adducted, and internally rotated, the elbows straight, the forearms pronated, the wrists and fingers flexed, and the thumbs on opposite hips. Adhering to the principle of normal timing, the distal component initiates the movement into D2F. The hands open, the forearms supinate, and the shoulders flex and externally rotate away from the body into the D2F pattern (Fig. 1B). The movement into flexion should occur in a diagonal line uncrossing in front of the body. Avoid the common error of keeping the arms too close to the body during movement and creating a circular motion or a windmill effect.

The *combining components* in the flexion motion (D2F) are: scapular elevation, adduction extend to the left in their respective diagonal patterns (Fig. 4B) The *trunk movement* that occurs with the UE asymmetrical flexion patterns is extension with rotation; trunk flexion with rotation occurs with UE asymmetrical extension patterns.

Activity: Standing; UE cross diagonal or reciprocal asymmetrical (CD) (RA)

Technique: Active movement

5

The cross diagonal pattern combines the two diagonal patterns with the limbs moving in opposite directions. One arm is positioned in D1E, the other in D2F (Figs. 5A, 5B). The arms cross in front of the body, one into D1F and the other in D2E. No movement of the trunk occurs in this combination as all accompanying trunk contractions are occurring simultaneously. This combination of extremity patterns can be used to promote trunk stability.

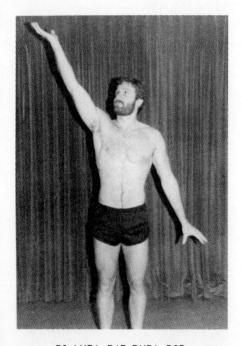

5A LUE in D1E; RUE in D2F.

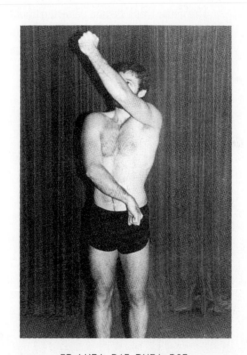

5B LUE in D1F; RUE in D2E.

6

Activity: Standing; trunk patterns—upper trunk extension-lift; upper trunk flexion-chop

Technique: Active movement

The upper trunk patterns which promote trunk extension or flexion in combination with rotation combine the asymmetrical patterns of the upper extremities. In these trunk patterns the arms are in contact with each other, one hand grasps the other forearm. This body-on-body contact closes the kinematic chain and seems to increase the activity of the trunk musculature.

The upper trunk extension pattern combines asymmetrical flexion patterns of the upper extremities and promotes upper trunk extension with rotation. To begin the movement both UEs are positioned in asymmetrical extension to one side, e.g., the right arm in D2E and the left arm in D1E. The left hand grasps the forearm of the right arm and the limbs move into the trunk extension pattern (Fig. 6A). The trunk, head, and neck move into extension with rotation. In the lift or **trunk extension pattern** the arm in the **D2 pattern leads** the movement, and the arm in the D1 pattern assists with the movement. The antagonistic movement combines bilateral shoulder extension and trunk flexion with rotation and is termed a reverse lift (Fig. 6B).

The upper trunk flexion pattern combines asymmetrical extension patterns of the upper extremities and promotes upper trunk flexion with rotation. The movement begins with the arms positioned in asymmetrical flexion to one side, e.g., the right arm in D1F and the left arm in

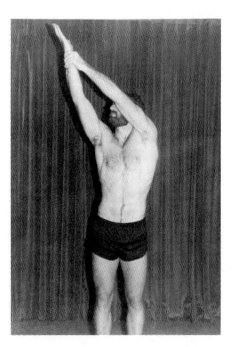

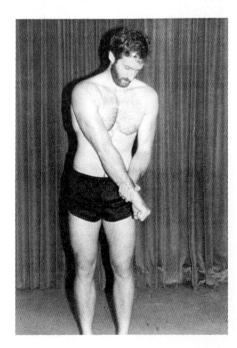

6A Shortened range of the trunk extensor movement.

6B Lengthened range of the trunk extensor movement.

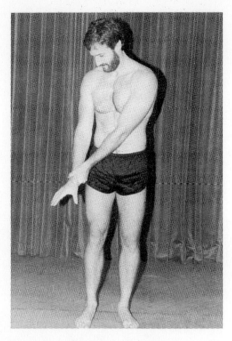

6C Shortened range.

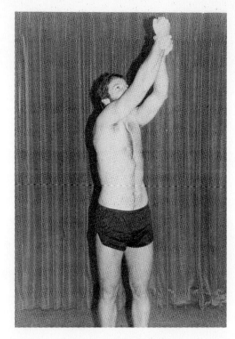

6D Lengthened range.

D2F. The left hand grasps the right forearm and both arms then extend into the trunk flexion movement (Fig. 6C). In the chop or **trunk flexion pattern** the **D1 pattern leads** the movement and the arm in the D2 pattern assists in the movement. The reverse or antagonistic pattern combines asymmetrical shoulder flexion and trunk extension with rotation and is termed a reverse chop (Fig. 6D).

Activity: Standing; lower extremity (LE) unilateral D1
Technique: Active movement

7

To practice this activity the therapists may need to hold onto each other's shoulders or onto a table for support. The right lower extremity (LE) is positioned in D1E (Fig. 7A); the hip is extended, abducted, and internally rotated, the knee extended, the foot plantarflexed and everted (the first toe is in contact with the floor). The leg flexes across the body either with the knee straight or moving into flexion (Fig. 7B).

The *combining components* in D1F are: pelvic protraction; hip flexion, adduction, external rotation; and ankle dorsiflexion with inversion. The *prime movers* of the hip and foot in D1F include the iliopsoas and the tibialis anterior.

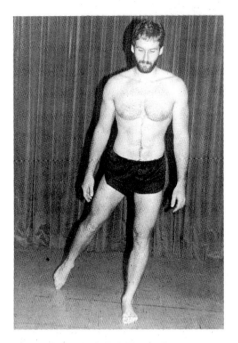

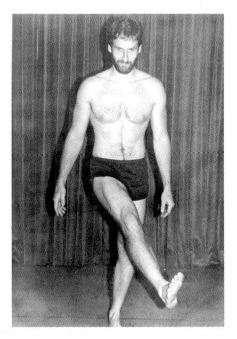

7A D1E.

7B D1F.

In D1E the movements are pelvic retraction; hip extension, abduction, internal rotation; an-kle plantarflexion with eversion (Chart 3). The *prime movers* in D1E include the gluteus medius and the peroneus longus. Note that this unilateral pattern performed in standing is a **static–dynamic** activity; the dynamic limb is the moving limb, the static limb is the weight-bearing limb.

CHART 3. Components of lower extremity patterns.

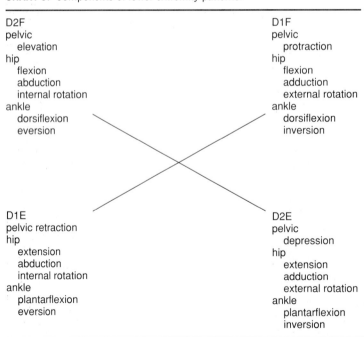

D2F
pelvic
    elevation
hip
    flexion
    abduction
    internal rotation
ankle
    dorsiflexion
    eversion

D1F
pelvic
    protraction
hip
    flexion
    adduction
    external rotation
ankle
    dorsiflexion
    inversion

D1E
pelvic retraction
hip
    extension
    abduction
    internal rotation
ankle
    plantarflexion
    eversion

D2E
pelvic
    depression
hip
    extension
    adduction
    external rotation
ankle
    plantarflexion
    inversion

Activity: Standing; LE unilateral D2
Technique: Active movement

8

The right LE is positioned in D2E with the hip extended, adducted, externally rotated, and crossed behind the left leg (Fig. 8A). The knee is straight and the toes are in contact with the floor; the foot is in plantarflexion and inversion. In D2F the leg is flexed, abducted, and internally rotated. The knee can remain straight or can flex with hip flexion (Figs. 8B, 8C).

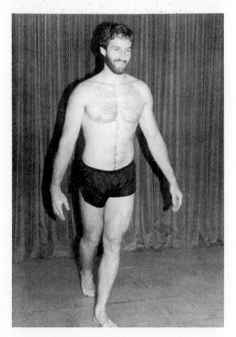

8A D2E.

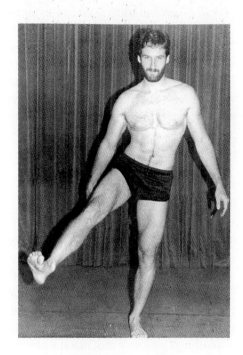

8B D2F (knee straight).

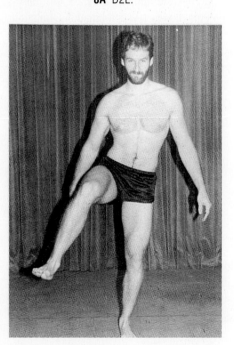

8C D2F (knee flexed).

D2E combines pelvic depression, hip extension, adduction, and external rotation with ankle plantarflexion and inversion (see Chart 3 on page 12). The *prime movers* in D2E include the gluteus maximus and the tibialis posterior.

The *combining components* in D2F are: pelvic elevation; hip flexion, abduction, internal rotation and ankle dorsiflexion with eversion. The *prime movers* at the hip and the foot in D2F include the tensor fasciae latae and the peroneus brevis. The D2F pattern incorporates hip flexion with ankle dorsiflexion and eversion, which is an important combination during advanced gait activities.

All of the limb patterns can be performed with the position of the intermediate joint, elbow or knee, varying using one of three motions: (1) the intermediate joint can flex with shoulder or hip flexion and extend with proximal extension; (2) it can remain straight throughout the movement; or (3) it can extend with shoulder or hip flexion and flex with shoulder or hip extension. The movement of the intermediate joint may be altered for specific therapeutic purposes and will be discussed in the section on extremity patterns.

9

Activity: Rolling
Technique: Active movement

The following rolling procedures are performed as active movements so that therapists can experience and observe the many combinations of movement patterns normally used to roll.

One group of therapists lies supine on the mats and rolls toward prone and back to supine. The other group observes the various normal combinations used in rolling. Some people initiate the movement with the head, some with the arm, others with the leg. Log rolling or segmental trunk rolling also may be observed. All of these combinations of movement occur in healthy individuals and may vary with movement repetition. The *prime movers* of rolling toward prone include the abdominals; the extremities flex and adduct across the midline. Patients with motor control deficits may be restricted to stereotyped movements or very few combinations. Initiation of movement from prone to supine requires activation of the trunk extensors. The groups of therapists should exchange places so that everyone has an opportunity to observe and experience the movements.

In the following procedures different combinations of upper extremity or upper trunk patterns are combined with the rolling movement to emphasize specific head, neck, and trunk movements. The lower extremity consistently moves in the D1 pattern.

10

Activity: Rolling; D1 UE; D1 LE
Technique: Active movement

Lying supine on the mat the therapist's upper and lower limbs are positioned in ipsilateral D1E (Fig. 10A). The activity is rolling toward prone but ending in the sidelying position. During the rolling activity the arm and leg flex and adduct across the body into the D1F pattern (Fig. 10B). The LE moves in mass flexion with the knee crossing the midline. When rolling back to supine,

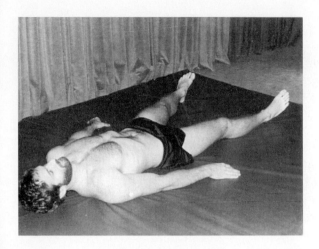

10A Beginning range.

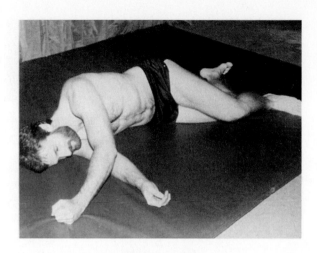

10B End range.

both the arm and leg move back into D1E. The trunk motions that accompany the extremity patterns were previously discussed.

Patients with a dominant asymmetrical tonic neck reflex (ATNR) or symmetrical tonic labyrinthine reflex (STLR) may have difficulty adducting the extremities across the midline or initiating the trunk movement.

Activity: Rolling; D2E UE; D1F LE

Technique: Active movement

11

In this activity the UE is positioned in D2F with the ipsilateral LE in D1E (Fig. 11A). When rolling toward sidelying the arm extends, adducts, and internally rotates down and across toward the opposite hip; the head and upper trunk flex and rotate. The LE, similar to the previously described activity, flexes and adducts in a mass D1 flexion pattern. In sidelying the UE and LE are crossed. The activity of rolling toward prone with this combination of extremity patterns facilitates total body flexion (Fig. 11B). The reverse movement to supine facilitates total body extension. Because the motion toward prone promotes flexion, it is very useful for patients who have total body extensor spasticity. In such cases the therapist assists the patient to roll toward prone then passively rolls the patient back to supine. When movement in one direction is emphasized, it is termed **unidirectional movement.** The phrase **reversing movements** is used when both directions are equally emphasized.

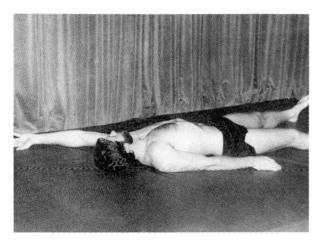

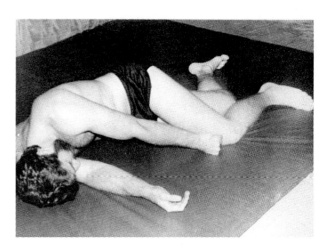

11A Beginning range.

11B End range.

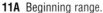

12

Activity: Rolling with upper trunk flexion and upper trunk extension
Technique: Active movement

Upper trunk patterns can be performed with the contact at the elbows, forearms, or hands, which progressively increases the length of the lever arm and number of joints involved.

Rolling to sidelying can be enhanced by the trunk flexion pattern or its reverse motion. The trunk flexion with rotation motion can be used to promote rolling when the major problem is either increased extensor tone as previously discussed or trunk flexion weakness. For example, a paraparetic with weak abdominals may be able to roll toward prone more easily when performing the upper trunk flexion pattern (Figs. 12A, 12B). A hemiplegic patient who demonstrates unilateral UE weakness or neglect may be able to roll from supine toward the less affected side by holding onto the involved limb and using the reverse chop pattern. This combination incorporates crossing of the midline of the upper extremities and movement of the involved limb into

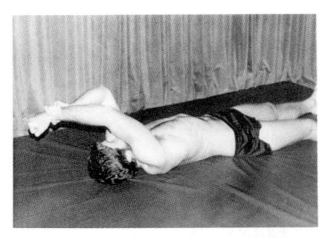

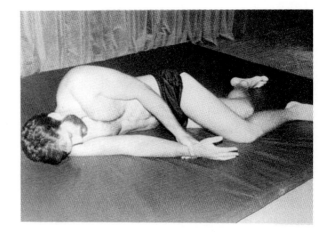

12A,B Upper trunk flexion (chop).

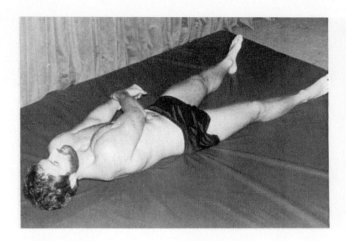
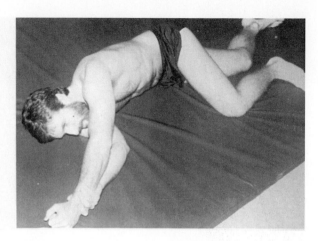

12C,D The reverse of the trunk flexion motion (reverse chop).

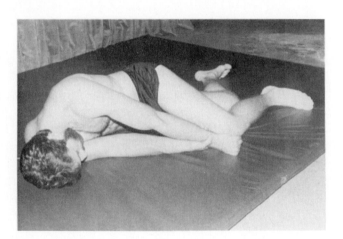
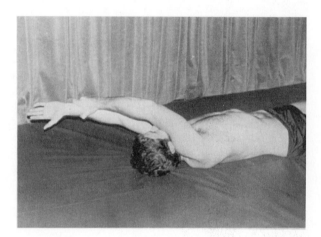

12E,F Upper trunk extension (lift).

shoulder flexion with adduction to avoid reinforcement of synergistic movements (Figs. 12C, 12D). Although rolling toward supine is not usually as difficult as rolling toward side lying and prone, this functional movement can be facilitated with a pattern that enhances extensor tone (Figs. 12E, 12F).

Study Questions

1. Which patterns promote shoulder flexion with abduction and external rotation?
2. List the prime movers of each joint in each pattern.
3. You are leading a group exercise program that includes patients with increased thoracic kyphosis and others with generalized trunk stiffness. Which movement patterns would be appropriate to address these impairments? Which limb and trunk motions occur with each pattern of movement?

part two

Procedures

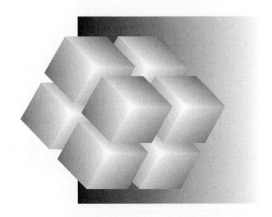

Mat Procedures

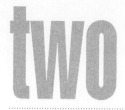

Chapter Outline

Key Terms

Mobility
Stability
Controlled Mobility
Static–Dynamic
Skill
Dynamic Stability
Impairment
Parameter
Rhythmic Initiation (RI)
Hold Relax Active Motion (HRAM)
Shortened Held Resisted Contraction
  (SHRC)
Alternating Isometrics (AI)
Rhythmic Stabilization (RS)
Slow Reversal Hold (SRH)
Slow Reversal (SR)
Agonistic Reversals (AR)
Resisted Progression (RP)
Repeated Contractions (RC)
Tracking Resistance

The procedures, consisting of activities, techniques, and parameters, are grouped into rolling, prone, lower trunk, and upright progressions.

Within these progressions the activities, the postures and movement patterns are sequenced according to various principles. These principles include *decreasing the size of the base of support from large to small, increasing the height of the center of gravity or of the center of mass, increasing the number of joints involved and increasing the length of the lever arm.*

Treatment techniques are incorporated into the procedure to remediate the impairments that result in control deficits. The stages of control which are achieved with techniques are:

STAGES OF CONTROL

Mobility

ROM:	passive motion through full range
Initiation:	ability to initiate active motion

Stability

Muscle:	ability to hold an isometric contraction in shortened ranges
Postural	ability to maintain midline and weight-bearing postures

Controlled Mobility

Weight shifting:	ability to weight shift in weight-bearing postures encompassing both concentric and eccentric contractions
Rotation:	ability to control rotation around a longitudinal axis
Static–dynamic	ability to move between postures and to maintain and move within weight-bearing postures with reduced extremity support
	ability to control segmental-rotational motions
Skill	ability to perform functional tasks including activities of daily living and ambulation with normal timing, sequencing and coordination of movement, and to control counterrotational movement.

Strength and endurance are inherent components of each stage of control and encompass actin-myosin bonding, alpha-gamma coactivation, circulation, and nutrition. All are required to initiate and sustain the muscle and total body response.

The parameters pertain to the intensity, frequency, duration, and speed of the performance of the procedure. Parameters are chosen based on the patient's physiologic capability, the reactivity of the musculoskeletal or neural tissue, and motor learning requirements. The procedures as delineated in this text do not provide a detailed description of the parameters as they need to be individually determined for each patient. General principles include: *intensity levels below approximately 40% are chosen when stability and endurance are the goals; frequency is massed for short-term learning and distributed for long-term retention; speed is gradually increased as motor learning occurs to enhance functional carryover.* In planning treatment, procedures are selected and sequenced based on the functional outcome desired and the required muscle or movement responses necessary to achieve that outcome.

Accompanying each procedure in this text are the impairments for which the procedure would be appropriate. The activity and technique are subsequently described followed by the clinical purpose and treatment goals that can be achieved. Lastly, common problems in the application of the procedure are discussed.

Rolling Progression

ACTIVITIES

Supine
Sidelying
Rolling

FACTORS RELATING TO THE PROGRESSION OF ACTIVITIES

Biomechanical Factors

Base of support large
Center of gravity low
No weight-bearing joints
Lever arm can be altered
Resistance provided by gravity and manual contacts

Reflexive Factors

Tonic reflexes may resist trunk flexion and rolling
Righting reactions may assist rolling
Postural control needs minimized

Activity: Rolling; supine toward prone
Technique: Rhythmic initiation (RI); MC scapula and pelvis
Impairments: Decreased ability to initiate movement due to diminished voluntary activation; hypertonia; motor learning deficits; poor sensory feedback or deficient feed forward responses.

13

Description

The procedure begins in the sidelying position so that the patient does not have to overcome reflex influences and the effects of gravity in the supine position. The patient's uppermost UE can be positioned across the body with the hand on the opposite shoulder to reduce the tendency of the wrist to fall into hyperflexion on the mat. The uppermost LE is positioned in some flexion and adduction across the other leg. The therapist may be in a kneeling or heel sitting position either in front of or behind the patient. Patients who depend on visual cueing may perform the rolling activity more easily if the therapist is positioned in front. The therapist's position, however, must not prevent the patient from performing the full rolling motion.

The technique of RI begins with the therapist passively moving the patient from supine toward prone through small ranges of motion. Both the range of movement and the amount of patient effort are gradually increased as the therapist feels the patient relax. As the amount of patient effort is increased the amount of assistance provided by the therapist is decreased. The progression is from passive to active assisted to slightly resisted movement, from slow to faster motion, and from midrange to full range movement. The minimal amount of resistance given at this mobility stage is termed **tracking resistance** and is provided to help the patient sustain the active muscular contraction by the additional tactile cues and the enhanced proprioceptive

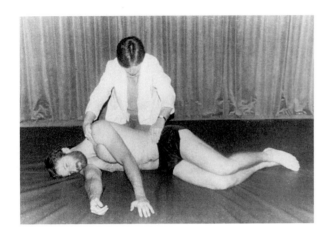

13A RI: Resistance to abdominals.

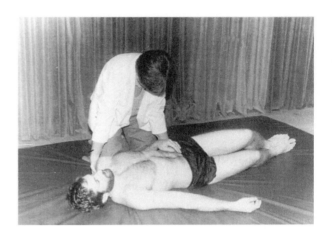

13B RI: Resistance to extensors.

feedback. One manual contact (MC) is positioned proximally on the scapula, to adequately resist or assist the trunk and to prevent any strain on a painful or flaccid shoulder. The other MC is on the pelvic crest to guide the lower trunk movement. To assist the rolling motion, MCs can be placed simultaneously on both sides of the joint. During the resistive phase, however, the MCs are alternately positioned on one side of the trunk in the direction of movement to provide minimal resistance to that movement (Figs. 13A, 13B). The verbal commands throughout the procedure should be soothing and should progress from "relax and let me move you" (passive phase) to "move slowly back and forth, move with me" (active assisted) to "roll forward and back and move into my hands" (tracking resistance).

Purpose/Treatment Goals

The purposes of the procedure are to: improve the patient's ability to initiate rolling from supine toward prone, decrease hypertonia, and improve motor learning.

The decrease in tone that may occur with this technique may be due to the rhythmical vestibular stimulation and the rotational joint movement. The technique was originally designed to balance tone in patients with Parkinson's syndrome but is appropriate for any patient with hypertonia. Patients with aphasia or apraxia also may benefit from this procedure. RI, because of its repetitive and rhythmic movement, promotes feedback and learning of the motor activity. The tracking resistance provided in this technique may facilitate the contraction and improve peripheral feedback by maintaining a slight external stretch on the muscle.

To protect the wrist extensors and shoulder flexors from being overstretched, the uppermost UE can be maintained in the position described above or at the patient's side. To incorporate UE motion into the rolling activity, the reverse chop trunk pattern or the "prayer position," i.e., hands clasped with shoulders flexed and elbows extended, may be used.

Problems with Application

Therapists may move the patient too quickly during the passive phase and thus facilitate an increase in tone instead of promoting relaxation. Therapists also may have difficulty with the placement of MCs during the transition from passive, to active assisted, to resisted movement. Remember that in the passive phase, MCs are on both sides of the body. As excessive tone diminishes and the patient begins to perform the activity, MCs are placed on the side of the body toward which the patient is moving to provide tracking resistance. This transition of MCs is essential for the therapist to properly control the procedure.

Activity: Rolling; supine toward prone
Technique: Hold relax active motion (HRAM); manual contacts scapula and pelvis
Impairments: Weak abdominals (less than 3/5) and a decreased ability to initiate movement.

14

Description

This procedure is used with patients who cannot initiate rolling from the lengthened range or who cannot sustain the contraction through full range because of weakness or hypotonia. To determine the need for this procedure the therapist applies a quick stretch to the trunk flexors, abdominals, to facilitate the rolling movement from supine to prone. The patient with musculature graded as 1 or 2/5 will respond minimally. The muscles may not respond adequately to the stretch because of a lack of stretch sensitivity or because of insufficient actin-myosin bonding. To enhance the response the muscles (or movement pattern) are positioned in or near their shortened range. The activity of rolling toward prone would begin in the sidelying position (Fig. 14A). In this shortened position an isometric contraction is applied to facilitate the internal stretch of the abdominal muscles and enhance cross bridge formation before facilitating the response from more lengthened ranges.

To perform this procedure the therapist kneels behind the patient and places MCs on the scapula and the pelvis. In the sidelying position, shortened range, an isometric contraction of the abdominals is gradually elicited by manual resistance until a maximum contraction is achieved. Remember that the muscle grade is 2/5 and therefore resistance must be minimal. The patient is then told to relax and is passively but quickly brought to supine, the lengthened range, where a quick stretch is applied to the abdominals (Fig. 14B). Coinciding with the quick stretch is the command to roll over. The subsequent contraction receives tracking resistance, or assistance if needed, to facilitate a response. The commands are "hold" in the shortened range then "relax," as the patient is quickly returned to the lengthened range; the final command is "roll back to you side," as stretch and resistance are applied to the contraction (Fig. 14C). The technique is then repeated.

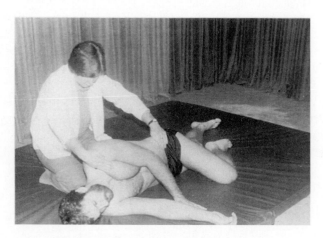

14A HRAM: Hold in shortened range.

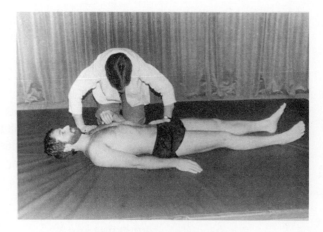

14B HRAM: Stretch in lengthened range.

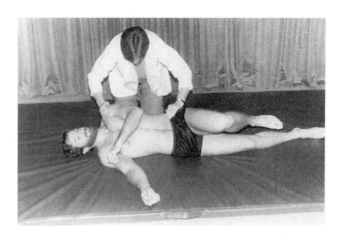

14C HRAM: Tracking resistance through range.

Purpose/Treatment Goals

The purposes of the procedure are to promote the mobility stage of control by enhancing the patient's ability to initiate movement and to sustain an active isotonic contraction throughout the range.

The purposes of the isometric contraction in the shortened range are to recruit gamma motor neurons to develop internal stretch in the muscle spindles and to enhance actin-myosin bonding. Patients for whom this procedure may be indicated are those with hypotonia, e.g., Guillain–Barré syndrome or muscular dystrophy.

HRAM is considered a unidirectional technique in that only one direction of the movement is emphasized. Because its purpose is to enhance active motor responses, the command to "roll" should be stressed.

If in the lengthened range, supine, the facilitated contraction is still not sufficient to overcome the resistance of body weight and gravity, assistance to the rolling movement is provided. The therapist must carefully grade the amount of assistance or resistance so that the abdominal contraction is facilitated, not overcome. The response anticipated is a more brisk, stronger contraction or an ability to sustain the contraction through greater ranges.

Problems with Application

Therapists frequently ask the patient to actively roll back to supine or resist the rolling activity backward rather than returning the patient passively to this position. The purpose of the procedure is to facilitate the abdominals. Active contraction of the extensors may lead to reciprocal inhibition of the abdominals that is counterproductive to the purpose of the procedure.

Therapists may have difficulty with the timing of the procedure. The patient must be returned to the lengthened range quickly to take advantage of the spindle sensitivity that may be developed in the shortened range.

The command to roll should be dynamic to further enhance the abdominal contraction.

Summary

Two procedures to improve the mobility stage of motor control during rolling have been performed with different techniques: (1) RI—to decrease tone and improve the initiation of movement in patients with hypertonia or problems with motor learning and (2) HRAM—to improve the active contraction of muscles and the ability to initiate motion and sustain the movement throughout the range in patients with weakness or hypotonia.

The *functional outcome* of these two procedures is that the patient will be able to initiate and sustain the rolling movement necessary for bed mobility. Because rolling toward prone is usually more problematic than rolling toward supine, this direction has been described. Modifications can be made to alter the direction. Emphasis can be placed on either upper or lower trunk segments as needed.

	Mobility	Stability	Controlled Mobility	Skill
Sidelying	Rhythmic initiation	Shortened held resisted contraction		
	Hold relax active motion	Alternating isometrics Rhythmic stabilization		

The following three procedures are used to develop trunk stability in the sidelying position. Stability, as used in this text, is the ability of muscles acting as functional extensors to **hold** an isometric contraction in the shortened range, and the ability to **maintain** either midline or weight-bearing positions. Static balance in the posture is promoted at this stage.

Activity: Sidelying; modified pivot prone

Technique: Shortened held resisted contraction (SHRC); MC as needed

Impairments: Weakness of head, neck, trunk extensors, or scapular stabilizers.

15

Description

Stability procedures begin with holding an isometric contraction of the postural extensors in their shortened range. During development the child may perform muscle holding in the pivot prone–prone extension posture before maintaining weight-bearing postures. However, many patients, particularly adults, cannot assume or maintain the pivot prone position for various reasons such as compromised cardiopulmonary status, marked weakness in the back extensors, decreased mobility (ROM) in the upper and lower back and hips, or dominant tonic reflexes. For these patients isometric holding can be performed in sidelying, supine, or sitting positions.

The therapist is behind the patient, who is in sidelying. MCs are placed on the part of the body to be isometrically resisted: the head, for patients with poor head control (Fig. 15A); the scapula, for the rhomboids and middle trapezius (Fig. 15B); the arm, for the posterior deltoid (Fig. 15C); the wrist, for the triceps (Fig. 15D); the lower back or pelvis, for the lower trunk extensors (Fig. 15E); or the thigh, for the gluteus maximus and medius. This technique promotes a gradual increase in isometric tension in the postural extensors. To enhance control in the postural extensors the contraction may be held for approximately 10 seconds; to improve muscle endurance the contraction is sustained for longer durations. The verbal commands are "hold" or "don't let me push you," not "push against me." The former produces an isometric hold; the latter an isometric push. Where appropriate, approximation can be applied to enhance the isometric contraction.

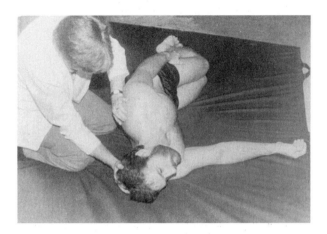

15A SHRC: MC head and scapula.

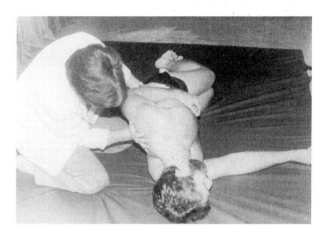

15B SHRC: MC scapula.

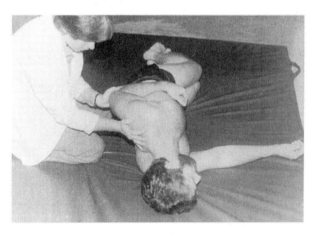

15C SHRC: MC scapula and elbow.

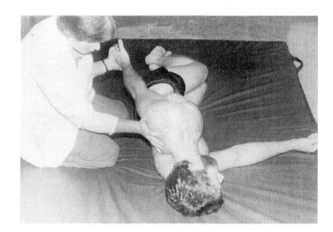

15D SHRC: MC scapula and hand.

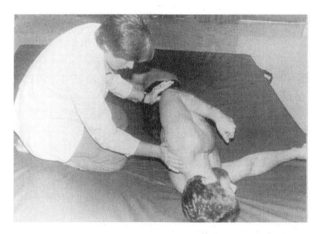

15E SHRC: MC scapula and pelvis.

Purpose/Treatment Goals

The purposes of the procedure are to promote a gradual increase and sustained isometric contraction of the postural extensors in the shortened range followed by a controlled gradual relaxation of the contraction, and to prepare the patient for weight-bearing activities.

The SHRC should be applied to the postural extensor muscles in shortened ranges to avoid the inhibition that may occur when extensor muscles contract in lengthened ranges. The contractions should not exceed 40 to 50 percent of maximum to activate primarily the type I muscle fibers. The technique of a SHRC, promoting muscle stability in shortened ranges, is preliminary to the second stage of postural stability, maintaining midline or weight-bearing postures.

Patients with hemiplegia can be positioned in a sidelying position on either side. If the involved limbs are lowermost, an increase in sensory stimulation to that side may occur from the body weight, and the lateral trunk can be elongated. Special care must be taken, however, to position the scapula so that the posture is not causing or aggravating a painful shoulder condition. If the involved limbs are uppermost, then the limbs can be positioned so as to discourage synergistic or spastic patterns, for example, the leg can be placed in mass flexion with adduction or in an advanced combination with hip extension and knee flexion.

Problems with Application

Patients with hypertonia may have difficulty modulating the intensity of the isometric contraction. In these situations the increase of muscle tension facilitated by the therapist's resistance must be graded carefully, followed by a gradual relaxation of the contraction. If the response is greater than desired, even with this modification, procedures to reduce hypertonia may need to precede this technique. (See Procedure 13, Activity: Rolling; Technique: Rhythmic initiation [RI].)

When facilitating muscle holding in patients with hypotonia, the therapist may need to begin with the muscles positioned on a slight external stretch to reduce the slack on the muscle spindle that occurs in the shortened range. In addition to approximation, facilitory inputs, such as overflow from intact segments or vibration may enhance the muscle response.

Activity: Supine flexion
Technique: Assist to position and holding of the posture; MC as needed
Impairments: Decreased abdominal strength; imbalance of trunk flexor and extensor strength; decreased righting reactions in supine.

16

Description

Supine flexion facilitates holding in the oblique abdominal muscles. The patient is positioned in neck and trunk flexion. The upper extremities may be adducted across the chest and the lower extremities are in mass flexion. The therapist assists the patient into trunk flexion by placing MCs under the head or the scapula. Adults may enhance upper abdominal strength with a sit-up and lower abdominal control with procedures in hooklying (see Procedure 39).

Purpose/Treatment Goals

The purposes of the procedure are to (1) develop holding in the abdominals, (2) facilitate righting reactions of the head and the trunk, and (3) promote a balance between trunk flexion and extension. This procedure is primarily performed with infants and small children or with adults with excessive extensor tone. The procedure can be performed in either supine or sidelying.

17

Activity: Supine; cervical, thoracic, lumbar, hip or knee extension

Technique: Shortened held resisted contraction (SHRC); MC as needed

Impairments: Decreased muscle stability or muscle endurance in any of the postural trunk extensors, gluteals, or quadriceps.

Description

The patient is positioned supine with a pillow under the head and another pillow under the knees. To teach the patient how to perform the technique, the therapist's MCs may be under the head, under the elbows, or under the knees. The therapist resists the isometric extensor contraction maintaining the amount of patient effort at or below approximately 40%. Verbal commands may be "push your head into the pillow," "push your elbows into the bed or mat and raise your chest," "push your knees into the pillow and lift your hips about one inch off the surface" (Fig. 17A). To indicate the duration of effort suggestions may be "hold the contraction for 3 to 5 breaths" or "hold the position for 5, to 10, to 30 seconds."

Purpose/Treatment Goals

The purpose of this procedure is to increase muscle stability and endurance of the cervical, thoracic, lumbar, hip and knee extensors in preparation for postural stability. Because some of these movements are assisted by gravity they are less difficult than trunk and limb extension performed in the prone position. In supine, the contraction can be performed bilaterally in con-

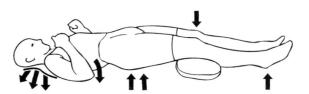

17A SHRC: Trunk and limb extension.

trast to the unilateral effort that occurs in sidelying. This is an exercise, which can be easily incorporated into the patient's independent and home program.

Patients with dysfunction in the cervical, thoracic, and lumbar spinal regions commonly have complaints of muscle fatigue, pain, or "burning." These symptoms may be indicative of poor muscle endurance or stability. This stability procedure can be included very early in a treatment sequence to begin to improve muscle control. In addition, if the primary problem is ligamentous or capsular in nature, improved muscle stability may help decrease the stress on these involved tissues. Improving muscle stability may also enhance proprioception that is required to enhance spinal alignment and correct posture.

Hip and knee extension can be promoted for patients with poor stability in these segments. To improve the simultaneous contraction of the gluteus maximus and gluteus medius a resistive band can be placed above the knees and the patient can push out against the band while extending the hips.

Problems with Application

Because the patient performs the procedure independently it is difficult to monitor the amount of effort. Having the patient breath during the isometric contractions helps ensure an aerobic effort. Patients with sacroiliac dysfunction may complain of pain if hip extension is excessive. The range can be decreased or the patient can learn to contract the gluteals without actually raising the hips.

Activity: Sidelying

Technique: Alternating isometrics (AI) progressing to rhythmic stabilization (RS); MC scapula and pelvis

Impairments: Decreased postural stability in the trunk; decreased ability to sequentially or simultaneously contract the trunk extensors and flexors; imbalance of trunk flexors and extensors.

18

Description

The second stage of stability is the ability to maintain midline or weight-bearing postures and may be initially promoted in sidelying with the techniques of AI and RS. In sidelying, the trunk is positioned in midrange. To increase the patient's base of support (BoS) the uppermost arm and leg may be positioned in flexion in front of the patient. If the patient is a hemiplegic, the upper and lower extremities can be positioned to reduce associated reactions. For example, the shoulder can be flexed to 90 degrees and adducted, and the elbow, wrist, and fingers can be extended. The hip and the knee may be flexed, or the hip positioned in extension with the knee flexed. To increase the challenge to trunk control, the progression of difficulty would be to gradually decrease the support offered by the extremities.

When the patient can perform a SHRC, as promoted with Procedure 15, the techniques of AI and RS can be applied. AI promotes sequential isometric contractions in the trunk flexors and extensors; RS promotes simultaneous contractions in these muscle groups.

The therapist may be positioned behind or in front of the patient. To initiate AI, MCs are positioned posteriorly on the scapula and the pelvis. A gradual increase in isometric tension is developed in the back extensors, which are now positioned on slight stretch compared to the pivot prone posture (Fig. 18A). MCs are smoothly altered (a sliding motion) onto the anterior surface of the body (Fig. 18B). Without allowing relaxation, resistance is applied to promote an isometric contraction of the flexors. Once the patient can perform the alternating isometric con-

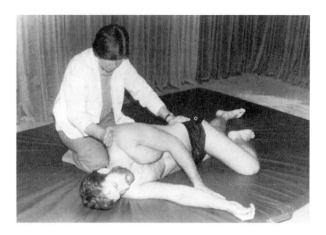

18A AI: Holding of extensors.

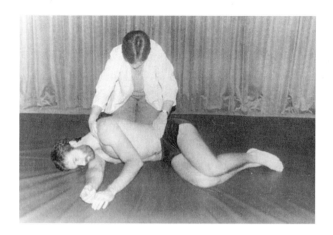

18B AI: Holding of flexors.

tractions (AI) with a gradual increase and decrease in intensity and a smooth transition between antagonists occurs, RS can be applied. The transition from the technique of AI to RS is made by the therapist switching one MC to the extensor surface of the trunk while the other MC remains on the flexor surface (Fig. 18C). Similar to AI, the technique of RS incorporates a gradual buildup and release of isometric tension with smooth transitions between the contractions. No relaxation is allowed during the transitions of resistance. The verbal commands during both techniques are "hold, don't let me move you." If, however, the patient has difficulty holding with one body part, commands can be directed specifically to that part, e.g., "don't let me move your hip forward or backward."

Purpose/Treatment Goals

In this sidelying position the techniques of SHRC, AI, and RS are performed to develop stability in the trunk and proximal joints.

SHRC initially develops muscle stability in the postural extensors so that when the muscle is subsequently positioned in a more lengthened range or when resistance is increased as occurs in weight-bearing postures such as sitting, the muscle may be able to cope with the added inhibitory influences of maintained stretch and resistance. AI may need to be performed before

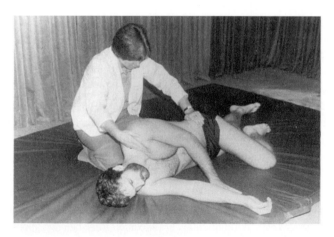

18C RS.

RS can be achieved. AI teaches the patient to alter isometric contractions. RS, which promotes postural stability, is the goal of the stability techniques. For patients with decreased stability in the upper trunk and scapula, MC can be positioned on the scapula and thorax. Stability in the lower trunk can be emphasized by altering MC to the pelvis and thorax or the pelvis and waist. Specific segmental stability can be promoted with MC on a specific spinous process and the pelvis. For example, patients with low back pain may have poor stability in the trunk muscula-ture. Total body stability with contacts on the scapular and pelvis can be followed by lower body stability with contacts positioned more closely to promote segmental stability. As more specific control is desired the amount of resistance is decreased to help localize the response.

Problems with Application

To perform these techniques correctly, the therapist changes resistive forces to either side of the joint or body part by altering pressure from the heels of the hands to the fingers. The use of a lumbrical grip (MCP flexed, PIP and DIP extended) may reduce the tendency to resist only with the finger tips. The MCs may have to slide from anterior to posterior surfaces if the body part is large. When altering resistance, the therapist should not lift the MCs; continuous contact is desired to facilitate stability.

Verbal commands are "hold, don't let me move you," or "don't let me push you forward or back." Therapists will often incorrectly say "push against me." For these stability techniques the desired contraction is an isometric hold, not an isometric push–pull. Being specific with verbal commands will help to promote a graded, controlled contraction.

The body mechanics of the therapist are important. If the patient is on a mat, the therapist kneels behind the patient; if the patient is on a table, the therapist can stand in front of or behind the patient. MCs can be placed on the scapula and the pelvis positioned closer together to focus on more segmental control. With the therapist's elbows near full extension, resistance can be provided by using body weight and trunk musculature. This results in smoother and more con-trolled application of resistance and provides the therapist with better leverage and body me-chanics.

Controlled mobility is the next stage of control and encompasses weight shifting in weight-bearing positions or total trunk rotation. Log rolling around the longitudinal axis is controlled mobility in the sidelying position. Static–dynamic procedures are usually an interim step be-tween the controlled mobility and the skill stages of control. In weight-bearing postures static–dynamic procedures are performed with one extremity moving while the other limbs are weight-bearing; in sidelying, static–dynamic trunk movements are segmental movements and occur when either the upper or the lower trunk holds as the other segment moves.

	Mobility	Stability	Controlled Mobility	Static Dynamic	Skill
Sidelying;			Slow reversal hold	Slow reversal hold	
log rolling			Slow reversal	Slow reversal	
segmental					
motions				Guided movement	

19

Activity: Sidelying; upper trunk rotation (UTR), lower trunk rotation (LTR)

Technique: Slow reversal hold (SRH); MC scapula and pelvis

Impairments: Imbalance of forward and backward rotation of the upper or lower trunk; imbalance of scapular motions; decreased pelvic rotation.

Description

Depending on the patient's impairments, either log rolling or segmental movements may be performed first. For students and some patients, teaching or performing the "part" or segmental motion, before the "whole" or log rolling may be easier. However, if tonic reflexes dominate or righting reactions are not well developed, segmental motions may be difficult. If the patient is unable to isolate the segmental movements of the trunk, the therapist may either return to the technique of RI (Procedure 13) or may need to promote log rolling before these segmental movements can be accomplished.

To perform segmental upper trunk movements, the therapist places one MC on the scapula; the other MC stabilizes the pelvis. The upper trunk is passively rotated forward and backward to allow the patient to experience the movement and to allow the therapist to feel the normal range for that movement. The movement performed can be upper trunk rotation or more specifically scapular movement in straight planes or in a diagonal direction.

The technique of SRH begins with a quick stretch in the lengthened range of the upper trunk flexion or extension motion. The contraction facilitated by this stretch is resisted into the shortened range where an isometric contraction is resisted (Fig. 19A). The isometric hold is followed by a quick stretch in the opposite direction to the antagonistic muscles. The isotonic contraction promoted by this stretch is resisted into the shortened range where an isometric contraction is performed (Fig. 19B). The reversing contractions are repeated a few times to promote a smooth reversal of antagonists. Resistance may be increased with each reversal.

To specifically emphasize the scapula rather than the upper trunk, the technique of SRH can be applied to the two diagonal patterns of the scapula. The scapular pattern in D1F combines elevation, abduction, and upward rotation (Fig. 19C) and D1E combines depression, adduction, and downward rotation (Fig. 19D). The *prime movers* include the serratus anterior, D1F, and the rhomboids and middle trapezius, D1E. In the D2F pattern, the scapular movement is elevation,

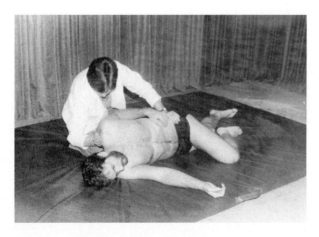

19A SRH: Stretch in lengthened range.

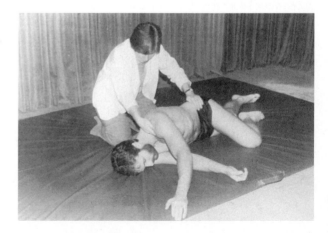

19B SRH: Holding in shortened range.

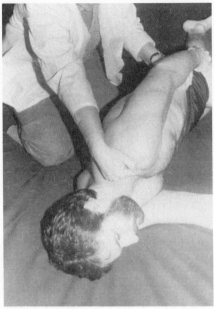

19C D1F.

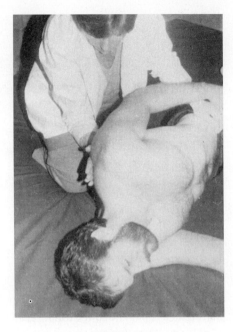

19D D1E.

adduction, and upward rotation (Fig. 19E), and in D2E the movement is depression, abduction, and downward rotation (Fig. 19F). The *prime movers* include the trapezius in D2F and the pectoralis minor in D2E. Frequently the progression of movements is from trunk rotation to the individual scapular patterns.

To shift emphasis from the upper trunk to the lower trunk or pelvic movement, the therapist is repositioned near the patient's hips to better resist the movement. The movement performed can be lower trunk forward or backward rotation or the pelvic motion that occurs in the

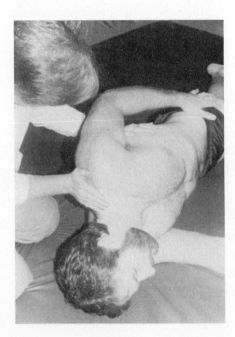

19E D2F.

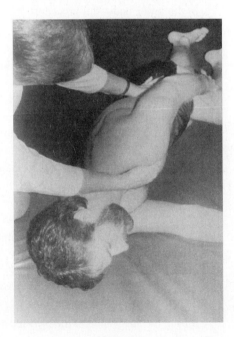

19F D2E.

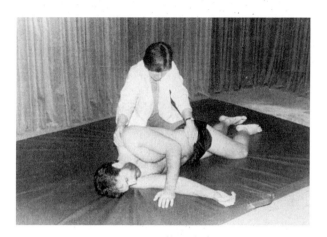

19G Resistance to abdominals in shortened range.

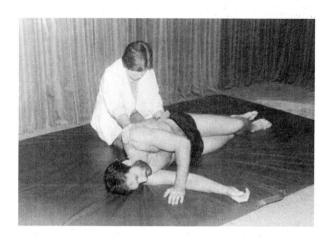

19H Resistance to pelvic extension.

D1 pattern, forward rotation with elevation. After passively moving the pelvis forward and backward to determine the lower trunk range, the pelvis is passively rotated back into the lengthened range of the abdominals and a quick stretch to these muscles is applied. As with the upper trunk movements, the contraction that follows is resisted into the shortened range where an isometric contraction is performed (Fig. 19G). Quick stretch and resistance are then applied to the antagonistic back extensor muscles (Fig. 19H) and the technique continued.

Purpose/Treatment Goals

The purposes of the procedure are to promote a smooth, coordinated, controlled reversal of antagonistic movements; enhance body-on-body reflex reactions by promoting segmental trunk rotational movement; and strengthen trunk flexors, extensors and rotators, and the scapular muscles. These segmental motions are preparatory for the trunk counterrotation that occurs during gait. As control is gained, the speed of the contractions can be increased.

In the lower body, the procedure may be performed to improve the lower trunk rotation and to strengthen the lower abdominals. Rotation can be performed in isolation or combined with elevation in the D1 pattern.

The technique of SRH with gradually increasing resistance will enhance the strength of the muscles. For those patients needing strengthening of the lower abdominals, e.g., patients with low back dysfunction, the progression of contractions is from isometric (AI, RS) to isotonic (SRH, repeated contractions [RC]). In the sidelying position the leg can be positioned in extension so that the shortened range of the hip flexor muscles is not reinforced. For these patients rotation of the lower trunk may be appropriately introduced in this nonweight-bearing position in which pressure on the disc and joint may be less than when the patient is in an upright posture. The range through which the patient moves may be gradually increased, termed increments of range.

For patients demonstrating a retracted pelvis in gait, segmental lower trunk rotation with emphasis on the forward rotational movement, protraction, is indicated. Hip flexion can be combined with forward pelvic rotation for patients having difficulty initiating the swing phase of gait (Figs. 19I, 19J). If the patient has an increase in lower extremity extensor tone, a mass flexion pattern of the leg is combined with the forward rotation of the pelvis. For this procedure, MCs are positioned on the pelvis and the thigh.

During the application of the SRH technique, the magnitude of the quick stretch applied in the lengthened range of the movement is slight. Healthy individuals have adequate stretch sen-

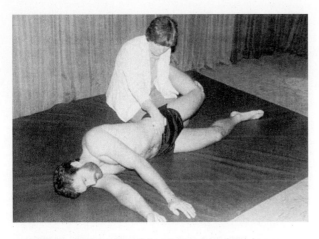

19I Hip flexion with pelvic rotation: Lengthened range.

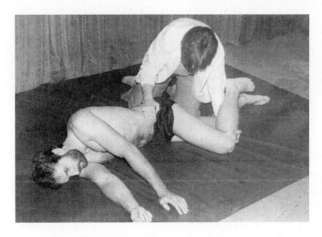

19J Hip flexion with pelvic rotation: Shortened range.

sitivity and do not require additional sensory input to facilitate movement. However, patients with weakened muscles or who lack muscle spindle stretch sensitivity usually require more external stretch to facilitate the movement.

Problems with Application

Many therapists apply excessive stretch and/or resistance. When these techniques are applied in excess, smooth reversals are difficult to attain. No relaxation should occur between the reversal motions and a smooth rhythm needs to be developed.

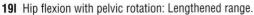

Activity; Rolling; supine toward prone, log rolling

Technique: SRH; MC scapula and pelvis

Impairments: Decreased ability to roll supine toward prone and back toward supine; weakness in abdominals and back extensors; dominance of tonic reflexes and decreased righting reactions.

20

Description

This procedure further promotes the patient's ability to independently roll, the controlled mobility stage of movement control. With the patient supine, MCs are positioned on the scapula and the pelvis and angled diagonally toward the midline. A quick stretch is applied to the abdominals and the isotonic contraction toward sidelying is resisted through the range of motion. In the shortened range an isometric contraction is performed. MCs then slide onto the posterior surface and a quick stretch is applied to the trunk extensors (Fig. 20A). As the patient moves back toward supine, the therapist's forearms supinate so that resistance can be provided throughout the range (Fig. 20B). In the supine position, MC can be altered onto the flexor surface to stretch the abdominals in two ways: (1) the therapist can keep the forearms supinated, slide the heels of the hands onto the flexor surface, and apply the quick stretch (Fig. 20C) followed by pronation of the forearms as the rolling movement is initiated (Fig. 20D) or (2) the therapist's forearms can be rotated into pronation with the fingers on the flexor surface and stretch and resistance applied with the fingers (Fig. 20E).

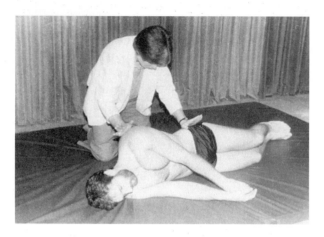

20A SRH: Quick stretch to the extensors.

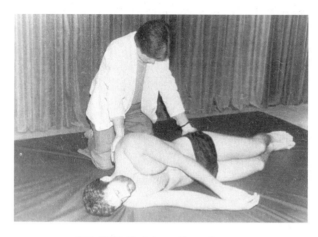

20B SRH: Resistance through range.

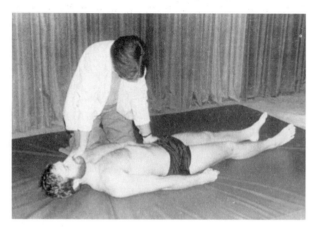

20C SRH: Stretch to the flexors.

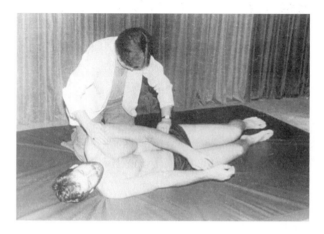

20D SRH: Resistance through range and holding in shortened range.

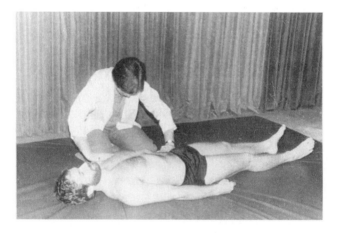

20E SRH: Stretch to the flexors.

Purpose/Treatment Goals

The purposes are to teach the functional activity of rolling; to enhance a smooth reversal of antagonists; to strengthen the trunk musculature; and to promote the controlled mobility level of movement control.

The rolling activity is supported by righting reactions and may help to integrate tonic reflexes. Log rolling can begin in either the supine or sidelying positions. If the patient has difficulty initiating movements from the full supine position, a pillow can be placed under the pelvis or the lower extremities can be crossed. The rolling activity can begin in sidelying if the patient cannot overcome the effects of gravity or influence of the tonic reflexes.

Problems with Application

The therapist may give too much resistance, thereby preventing a smooth reversal of movements. The transition between reversals may be difficult for the therapist and needs to be practiced. Regardless of the method chosen, the changing of MCs during the reversal of antagonists may be difficult because of the patient's size. As part of the learning experience the therapist must try to feel the unwanted relaxation between the reversal movements and make the proper manual adjustments.

Activity: Sidelying; counterrotation or adversive movements

Technique: Rhythmic initiation (RI); slow reversal (SR); MC scapula and pelvis

Impairments: Decreased trunk control; dominance of righting reactions.

21

	Mobility	Stability	Controlled Mobility	Skill
Sidelying; counterrotation				Slow reversal

Description

The patient is sidelying. The therapist, with MCs on the shoulder girdle and the pelvis, passively rotates the upper and lower body in opposite directions simultaneously.

The technique of RI progresses from passive, to active assisted movement, to tracking resistance, gradually increasing the speed and the range through which the movement occurs. During the passive and active assisted phases, both of the therapist's MCs are placed on both sides of the body. During the tracking resistance phase, however, MCs are placed on opposite sides of the body in the direction in which the patient is to move (Fig. 21A). To promote the desired response, a rhythmical movement needs to be maintained and the activity kept at a subconscious level. If one body part does not respond correctly, commands can be given to that part, "bring your shoulder forward, now roll it backward" or "roll your hip forward and backward."

Purpose/Treatment Goals

The purpose is to enhance counterrotation, the skill level of control in the trunk. This movement is needed for locomotion and skilled upper extremity function.

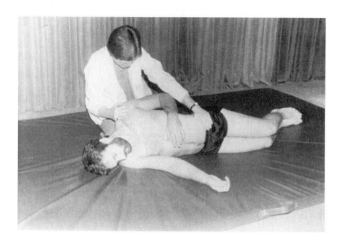

21A Trunk counterrotation.

Counterrotation is an advanced movement and is performed after segmental motions. Because strengthening is not a goal at this skill level of control, the technique of RI progressing to slow reversal is used and resistance kept to a minimum. Tracking resistance is applied to facilitate and guide the movement. Although this procedure is described near the beginning of the treatment sequence, it is usually performed toward the conclusion of rehabilitation to promote the trunk movements needed for a normal gait pattern. For many patients the movement of trunk counterrotation is difficult. To teach and enhance the motion the technique progresses from RI to SR.

Problems with Application

Therapists may have difficulty performing this procedure. Alteration of MCs between the assistive and the slightly resistive phase is difficult.

Therapists need to relax and find a rhythm. This procedure, perhaps more than most others, requires a great deal of practice to achieve a smooth, coordinated movement.

22

Activity: Supine or sidelying; breathing

Technique: Resisted movement; MC lateral chest wall

Impairments: Decreased chest wall mobility; decreased vital capacity or increased muscle tension.

Description

The therapist may need to intersperse the previous mat activities with procedures to facilitate breathing. With the therapist at the patient's side, MCs are placed on the chest wall in the angular direction of the ribs. As the patient breathes, the therapist feels the compliance of the rib cage. Following exhalation, a stretch is provided to facilitate chest expansion (Fig. 22A). Tracking resistance is applied during inspiration to provide the patient with feedback of the movement.

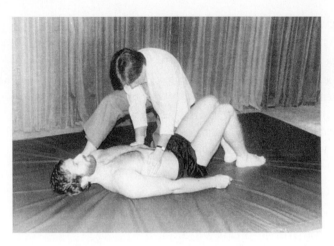

22A Quick stretch lateral chest wall.

Summary

We have concluded the procedures in the initial upright progression that include the activities of sidelying and rolling. In these activities, techniques were chosen to promote the stages of control. Mobility was achieved with the techniques of RI and HRAM. RI was used for patients with hypertonia to gain relaxation and to help initiate movement. HRAM was used to initiate movement in patients with weakness in the postural muscles. Stability was promoted with the techniques of SHRC, AI, and RS. SHRC was used to enhance muscle stability. AI was an intermediate technique to achieve RS and postural stability. Controlled mobility was gained with the technique of SRH during the activity of log rolling. Static–dynamic control was promoted with SRH to segmental movement. Skill was facilitated with SR to adversive trunk movements or counterrotation in sidelying.

Prone Progression

ACTIVITIES

Pivot prone
Prone on elbows
Prone on hands
Quadruped

FACTORS RELATING TO THE PROGRESSION OF ACTIVITIES

Biomechanical Factors

Base of support decreases
Center of gravity (mass) elevates from surface
Number of weight-bearing joints increases
Elongation of lever arm in both upper and lower extremities
Resistance provided by gravity to trunk extension, upper extremity flexion and lower extremity extension

Reflexive Factors

Tonic reflexes: The symmetrical tonic labyrinthine reflex reduces trunk and limb extensor tone and increases flexion. The symmetrical tonic neck reflex may increase upper extremity extension if the neck extends. These influences may be most evident in children who have central nervous system (CNS) pathology.

Righting reactions: The body on head and body on body reactions may enhance trunk extension in pivot prone and may assist in the assumption of prone on elbows and quadruped.

Postural control: Static stability is promoted as the postures are maintained; dynamic stability is enhanced as weight shifting is performed.

23

Activity: Pivot prone, prone extension

Technique: Shortened held resisted contraction (SHRC); MC scapulae or as needed

Impairments: Decreased muscle stability; decreased strength of trunk extensors below 3/5; decreased endurance of trunk extensors.

Description

Pivot prone, prone extension, the first posture of the prone sequence, is one of the postures where muscle stability can be developed in the deep one-joint postural extensors.

The patient is prone with the head in midline; the shoulders are extended and the elbows flexed. The patient may be positioned over a pillow, ball, wedge, or off the edge of a raised mat. The therapist is positioned by the side of the patient. If the patient needs to be assisted into the pivot prone posture, MCs are placed over the clavicles. Once in the position, assistance is withdrawn so that the patient maintains the position independently. To emphasize muscle stability in the lower trunk, MCs may be placed under the legs as the lower body extends or raises off the supporting surface.

Purpose/Treatment Goals

The purpose is to develop muscle stability in the postural extensors of the trunk and the limbs. Maintaining the isometric contraction in the shortened range may increase the muscle spindle stretch sensitivity in the postural muscles that is important for postural stability in all of the subsequent weight-bearing positions. The righting responses may be enhanced as the patient assumes and maintains this posture.

For patients with excessive thoracic kyphosis, improved posture may result from the increased control of the neck and back extensors, and the scapular adductors.

Muscle stability and improved muscle endurance in the lower body is essential before quadruped, sitting or other upright postures can be maintained.

Problems with Application

Patients may have difficulty assuming or maintaining this posture due to: decreased ROM and strength, diminished cardiopulmonary capacity, a dominance of tonic reflex influence, or a lack of righting reactions. In such cases extension can be promoted in modified pivot prone postures. These include sidelying, sitting, and supine.

Activity: Prone on elbows (P on E)

Technique: Assist to position; MC scapula

Impairments: Weakness of scapular, shoulder, and upper trunk muscles.

24

Description

The technique of assist to position is appropriate for patients who cannot independently assume the position; e.g., those with spinal cord injury. One means of assisting the patient is to position the patient in the prone position. The shoulders are flexed and abducted to about 145 degrees with the elbows flexed. With the arms positioned in this manner above 90 degrees they are more likely to fall under the shoulders when the upper body is lifted.

To help the patient move into the P on E posture, the therapist straddles the patient. To protect the therapist's back, one leg should be positioned in front of the other with the knees flexed. The therapist may prefer to assume the half-kneeling position or be by the patient's side. Using the flat part of the fingers, a lumbrical grip and not the finger tips, the MCs are placed over the clavicles away from the patient's neck (Fig. 24A). The patient receives the following instructions: "on the count of three you are going to come up onto your elbows. Ready? One, two, three, and up." The therapist assists the patient into P on E. Once in the position, approximation may be applied through the shoulders to help the patient stabilize in the posture. The therapist moves to the side of the patient in preparation for the performance of the stability techniques.

A modification of the procedure may be necessary for the patient with hemiplegia or trunk spasticity. For example, with MCs on the clavicles, the upper body is gradually extended and rotated off the mat. The patient's arms are then assisted forward into the P on E position.

Purpose/Treatment Goals

The purpose is to assist the patient (mobility) into the position when independent assumption of the position is not possible.

This procedure is most appropriate for children, for patients with spinal cord injury, or those with general body weakness such as Guillian–Barré. Modifications of the procedure can be made for other patients who would benefit from this posture and need assistance into the position.

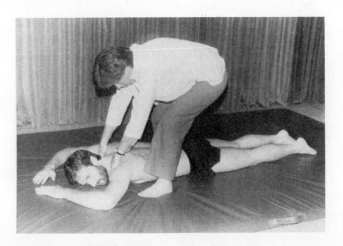

24A Initiation of the assist to P on E.

Problems with Application

If a patient who has dominant tonic reflexes hyperextends the head, the elbows may extend and the patient may come to the prone on hands position (STNR). Instruct the patient prior to the movement to bend the elbows as the P on E posture is assumed. The speed of the motion may need to be reduced if neck joint stability is compromised.

Some patients may find this P on E position difficult. Patients with hypertonia may exhibit an increase in upper extremity tone in the wrist and the finger flexors, forearm pronators, and shoulder internal rotators. Such an increase in tone indicates that the P on E posture is too stressful. When this occurs an alternate activity, such as sitting with UE weight bearing, should be used.

25

Activity: Prone on elbows

Technique: Alternating isometrics progressing to rhythmic stabilization (AI > RS)

Impairments: Decreased postural stability around the head, neck, upper trunk, scapulae, and shoulders; decreased ability to simultaneously contract the serratus anterior, middle trapezius, rhomboids, deltoid, and rotator cuff.

Description

The therapist half-kneels or heel sits by the side of the patient. With MCs on the shoulders, AI is performed by applying resistance to isometric contractions in the different directions of upper trunk movement. Resistance can be applied in a cephalocaudal direction (Figs. 25A, 25B), then in a medial-lateral direction (Figs. 25C, 25D). AI performed in a diagonal direction away from and toward the therapist combines the individual contractions just performed (Fig. 25E). AI can also be performed to the upper trunk in a clockwise-counterclockwise direction (Fig. 25F). When resisting in this direction, isometric resistance is focused on the upper trunk rotating around C7 and not on rotation of each scapula. The placement of MCs with AI alters with each direction of resistance. During cephalocaudal resistance, MCs are on the superior scapula, over the upper trapezius, and the heel of the hand is under the spine of the scapula. During diagonal and rotational resistance, the MCs are similar to the position just described but the direction of resistance is altered. For medial-lateral resistance, the MCs are on the lateral shoulders. When

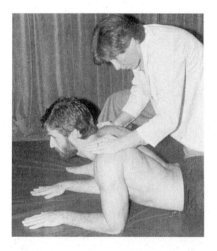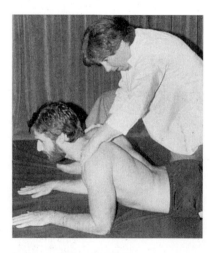

25A,B AI with resistance in an anterior posterior direction.

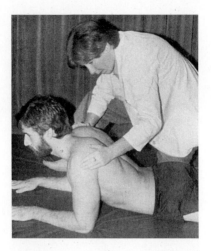
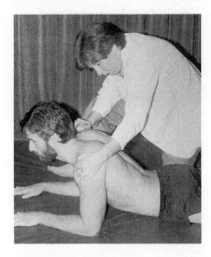

25C,D AI with resistance in medial lateral direction.

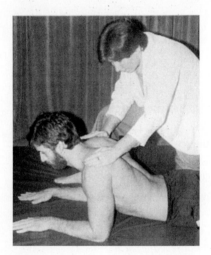
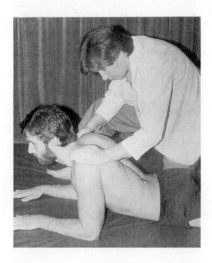

25E AI with resistance in a diagonal direction.

25F AI with resistance to upper trunk rotation.

the patient can perform AI in each direction and smoothly reverse isometric contractions, the technique can be progressed to RS.

RS facilitates simultaneous contraction on both sides of the supporting segments and combines resistance in all three directions of movement. One MC resists primarily the rotational component and the other resists primarily in the diagonal direction (Fig. 25G). In this P on E position, the MC closer to the therapist resists in the diagonal direction while the other MC provides rotational resistance. With no relaxation allowed, the other combination is resisted, i.e., pulling diagonally toward the therapist combined with the opposite rotational force. A smooth gradual switch of resistive forces is desired.

RS also can be applied with one MC on the head and the other on the shoulder to facilitate head and neck contraction. The MC on the head is placed on the crown of the head and diagonal resistive forces are alternately applied with the heel of the hand and the fingers. The resistance applied by the MC on the scapula is in the opposite direction of the same diagonal (Fig. 25H). With MCs placed either on the scapula or on the head and the scapula, approximation can be applied through the joints being resisted to facilitate proximal holding.

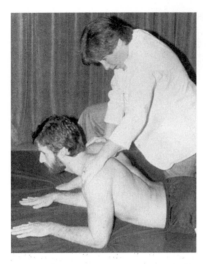

25G RS combining diagonal and rotatory resistance.

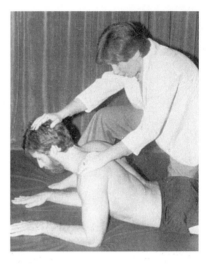

25H RS with MC on head and scapula.

Purpose/Treatment Goals

The purpose is to develop postural stability of the head and neck, the upper trunk, the scapulae, and the shoulders.

If the patient has difficulty controlling simultaneous isometric contractions AI can be used to teach, in a stepwise manner, the components of RS.

The procedure with MCs on the head and the shoulder is appropriate for patients with whiplash injuries when isometric contraction of the neck muscles is indicated. Proper positioning of the head and the neck in the midrange is emphasized. Excessive lower cervical forward flexion with head and upper cervical extension is discouraged.

For patients with shoulder pain, placement of MCs on the head and the uninvolved limb can be used as an indirect approach to promote isometric contractions in the painful limb. When MCs are not placed directly on the involved part, the term *indirect approach* is used.

Stability of the head and the neck is a prerequisite for proximal control in upright postures, as well as for speech and feeding. Thus, this stability procedure may be used to enhance head control and improve vital functions. If gravity or reflexes interfere with the facilitation of head and neck stability, the techniques can be applied in a less stressful, supported sitting position.

For hemiplegic patients this posture may be problematic: the elbow is flexed, the triceps are on prolonged stretch, and there is weight bearing on the triceps tendon. Because of the discomfort of maintaining the position, there may be increased abnormal tone in the UE. If an increase in tone is noted as the patient attempts to maintain the position, the posture may be considered too stressful and, as stated earlier, another activity, such as sitting with UE support, may be substituted (Procedure 50). An alternative is to place a pillow under the abdomen.

Problems with Application

The therapist may have difficulty differentiating between resistance to the rotational movements with AI and the combination of three planes of resistance with RS. In this very stable position, it may be difficult to feel the difference but when these techniques are applied in postures where the BoS is smaller, such as quadruped or sitting, the differences between the techniques may be more evident. At this time, it is important at least to understand that AI is resistance applied alternately in one or two directions or planes and RS is the simultaneous application of resistance in all three directions. To determine the direction of the resistive forces when applying AI to rotation, the analogy of rotating a steering wheel in a clockwise-counterclockwise direction, with C7 being the axis, may be helpful.

With both techniques the proper placement of MCs is important. Hands are placed whenever possible in a position so that they do not have to be lifted or moved during the change of resistance. Resistance should be provided with the heels of the hands in one direction and then with the fingers (not just fingertips) in the other direction. There should be no relaxation during the alterations of resistance during any of these stability techniques.

The resistance in RS should be repeated only three to four times as the patient may tend to hold their breath and increase intrathoracic pressure. If proper breathing patterns are encouraged and the resistance kept at a moderate intensity, the patient should not perform the Valsalva maneuver. For patients with acute cardiac or cranial involvement, these isometric contractions may be contraindicated.

Activity: Prone on elbows
Technique: Active movement
Impairment: Radicular LE pain

26

Maintaining the posture independently can be useful where increased lumbar extension is desired. For example, some patients with low back dysfunction may experience relief of radiating leg pain when lumbar extension is maintained. The therapist may need to ensure that the patient is using the upper extremities for support.

Activity: Prone on elbows; lateral weight shifting
Technique: Slow reversal hold (SRH); MC scapula or both shoulders
Impairments: Decreased scapular and shoulder strength; poor scapulohumeral rhythm; diminished postural responses in the upper body; dominant asymmetrical tonic neck reflex (ATNR).

27

	Mobility	Stability	Controlled Mobility	Skill
Prone on elbows	Assist to position	Alternating isometrics Rhythmic stabilization	Slow reversal hold through increments of range	

Description

Once stability in a posture is evident, the patient can be progressed to controlled mobility procedures. In P on E, a weight-bearing position, controlled mobility is accomplished by weight shifting. The technique of SRH is applied through increments of range, i.e., the movement occurs initially through small ranges then through larger excursions until the patient completes full range and all the upper body weight is shifted over the weight-bearing elbow.

The therapist is positioned at the side of the patient in a half-kneeling or heel sitting position. In the description below, the therapist is on the patient's right side. The left MC is placed on the lateral side of the left shoulder as the patient moves toward that side. A stretch to facili-

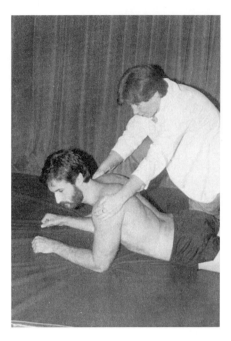

27A SRH: Lateral shifting left.

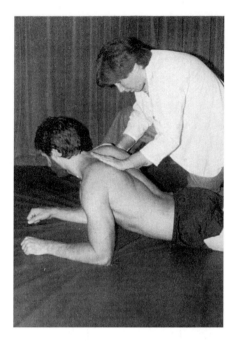

27B SRH: Lateral shifting right.

tate this lateral movement may be applied simultaneously with the command "move away from me." The patient shifts over the left elbow and resistance is applied mainly by the lateral hand. The right contact is positioned on the right clavicle or anterior shoulder as the patient laterally shifts away from the therapist. The lateral shifting motion is resisted and an isometric contraction is performed when the desired range is completed (Fig. 27A). To reverse the movement and shift toward the right, the right contact is repositioned laterally on the right shoulder, a slight stretch applied with this lateral MC, and the command "now move toward me" is given (Fig. 27B). The left contact is placed on the vertebral border of the left scapula. The MCs are moved sequentially; the MC on the lateral shoulder is positioned first followed by the other MC. The stretch is not applied to a specific muscle but rather to the lateral direction of movement. Rotation of the head in the direction of the lateral shift can increase both the range of movement and the amount of weight borne on each arm.

Purpose/Treatment Goals

The purposes are to: (1) promote integration of the ATNR, (2) develop dynamic postural control, (3) facilitate upper body lateral elongation, (4) promote the controlled mobility level of control, and (5) promote proximal dynamic stability.

Dynamic stability is a quality of movement. During skilled functional upper extremity movement in nonweight bearing, the proximal muscles provide dynamic stability to control the limb movement. Many patients excessively move the scapula during arm motions. A purpose of this procedure is to develop proximal dynamic stability to reduce the abnormal timing or sequencing of movement. This proximal control is gained more easily in weight-bearing positions where the body weight provides an approximation force to facilitate the stability component. Therefore, dynamic stability, needed during the skill stage of control is gradually developed during the performance of stability, controlled mobility, and static–dynamic procedures.

This activity is very appropriate for a patient who exhibits a dominant ATNR. Because the upper extremities are stabilized through weight bearing, abnormal upper extremity motions may be prevented during head rotation and the influence of the ATNR decreased.

The lateral reversals should be performed initially through small ranges. As the procedure continues, the range of excursion increases. If the patient has poor postural control responses, the gradual increase in weight shifting should help to develop dynamic balance.

For most patients, movement in the lateral direction may be sufficient to develop controlled mobility. For spinal cord injured (SCI) patients, expecially quadriplegics, inclusion of flexion and extension motions at the shoulder promoted by anterior-posterior weight shifting may help the patient progress to independent assumption of P on E. In addition, for these patients, arching of the upper trunk combined with neck flexion, a prerequisite for elevation in long sitting, can be accomplished in this P on E position. This upper body motion is the same as the motion in long sitting that elevates the hips and pelvis from the surface. This motion can be taught and practiced more easily in the P on E posture prior to long sitting.

Problems with Application

Therapists may have difficulty with the placement of MCs. The MC positioned on the lateral aspect of the shoulder is the one that provides the stretch and most of the resistance. The other MC can be alternately lifted if the therapist cannot coordinate its placement.

The verbal commands to move toward the right or left may be used but can be confusing to many patients. Other means of implying direction, i.e., "move toward me" or "move away from me," may be more appropriate.

Because the CoG is raised off the supporting surface, the magnitude of the stretch should be limited to prevent the patient from being displaced out of the BoS.

Graded resistance is provided to facilitate both the isotonic movement and the isometric hold.

....

Activity: Prone on elbows; D1 thrust

28

Technique: Slow reversal hold (SRH); MC scapula or shoulder (on static limb) and wrist (on dynamic limb)

Impairments: Weakness of scapular and shoulder muscles; decreased scapulohumeral rhythm.

Description

When the patient can weight shift through range, static–dynamic activities can be performed. Before performing this procedure the therapist may need to practice the D1 thrust pattern. The arms are positioned in D1 withdrawal, beginning with scapular adduction, shoulder extension, elbow, wrist, and finger flexion, and forearm supination; the fisted hand is in front of the shoulder (Fig. 28A). The D1 thrust combines scapular abduction, shoulder flexion, adduction, and external rotation, elbow, wrist, and finger extension, and forearm pronation (Fig. 28B).

For this static–dynamic procedure the patient is positioned in P on E. The therapist is diagonally in front of the patient opposite the dynamic limb. The patient's weight is laterally shifted onto one limb and the other upper extremity lifted from the supporting surface. One of the therapist's contacts approximates through the weight-bearing scapula and shoulder and this contact assists the patient with postural control in this weight-bearing position. The other MC is positioned on the wrist or forearm of the dynamic limb; it initially assists and then resists that arm through the D1 thrust–withdrawal pattern. Resistance to the thrust begins with a quick stretch in the lengthened range. The arm is guided forward into the shortened range where approximation is the primary resistive force during the isometric hold (Fig. 28C). A traction force

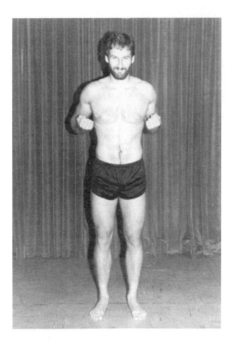

28A D1 withdrawal.

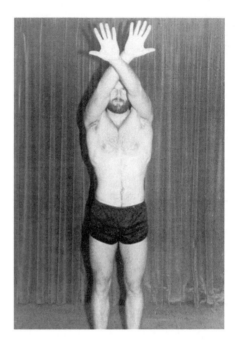

28B D1 thrust.

stretches the antagonist muscles of the withdrawal pattern followed by resistance through the range and an isometric contraction in the shortened range (Fig. 28D). The patient's eyes follow the movement of the dynamic limb to promote neck rotation or head crossing the midline and a greater excursion of motion.

Purpose/Treatment Goals

The purpose is to further enhance dynamic stability in the weight-bearing arm with the shoulder in 30 to 45 degrees of flexion.

The dynamic arm is the stronger or uninvolved limb. The amount of resistance applied to the dynamic limb depends on the strength and/or stability of the involved weight-bearing shoulder.

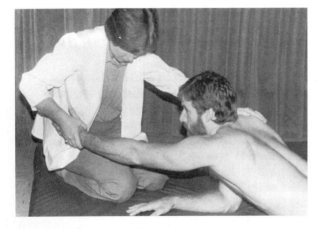

28C SRH: D1 thrust.

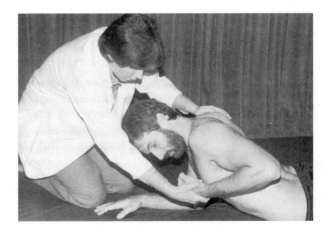

28D SRH: D1 withdrawal.

Dynamic stability is enhanced in the static limb as the dynamic arm is resisted. The movement of the dynamic limb and resistance to that limb alters the CoG and promotes dynamic balance responses in the weight-bearing limb. Dynamic stability is more advanced and requires more control than the static stability developed during the stability stage with the techniques of AI and RS. It is important that the dynamic arm flexes across the midline in the D1 thrust pattern. This adduction forces more weight onto the static limb, challenging the postural control of the scapular and glenohumeral musculature.

Problems with Application

The therapist may not be positioned on the diagonal and thus be unable to guide the dynamic arm through the correct movement. Incorrect positioning may actually interfere with the movement.

Too much resistance may be applied to the dynamic arm and stress the patient inappropriately or, conversely, the therapist may only assist the movement. The therapist observes the weight-bearing ability and scapular alignment in the weight-bearing arm. If the scapula lifts from the thorax or excessively abducts or rotates, the amount of manual resistance from the unilateral support may be too challenging. If this occurs, the therapist may need to decrease the excursion of the dynamic limb, decrease the amount of resistance, or return to the controlled mobility stage.

The skill level of control in this P on E position is crawling. Because this is not a functional activity for most patients, locomotion will not be practiced in this position.

....

Activity: Prone on hands
Technique: Active movement
Impairment: Decreased lumbar lordosis; pain radiating into the lower extremity; decreased stability in the upper extremity

29

Description

The patient may be assisted or may move actively into the prone-on-hands position.

Purpose/Treatment Goals

Patients who exhibit low back and leg pain may experience a decrease in symptoms as they move into and maintain the lordotic position.

Pediatric patients who have upper extremity weakness or instability can use this posture to increase upper quadrant stability.

Problems with Application

Patients with diminished respiratory capacity or cardiac insufficiency may not tolerate any prone posturing. The increased lordosis may be problematic for some patients with tightness in the hip flexors and would be contraindicated for those with spondylolisthesis.

30

Activity: Quadruped

Technique: Assist to position; MC on pelvis

Impairments: Decreased ability to independently assume the quadruped position.

Description

The independent assumption of a posture requires the controlled mobility level of control. Many patients can maintain a posture before they can assume the posture independently. In this procedure the patient is assisted into the position so that stability and initial weight-shifting activities can be performed in preparation for the independent assumption of the position.

The procedure begins with the patient positioned in P on E. The patient's knees may need to be slightly separated so that a sufficient BoS is provided in the quadruped position. Proper body mechanics of the therapist are stressed. The therapist straddles the patient's legs and the therapist's knees are flexed with one foot positioned in front of the other. With MCs on the patient's pelvis, the therapist alternately rotates and shifts each side of the patient's pelvis in a lateral and backward direction while the patient walks back on elbows (Figs. 30A, 30B). When the hips and the knees reach 90 degrees of flexion, approximation is applied through the hips (Fig. 30C). The upper extremities then can be assisted into the position of elbow extension with weight bearing on the hands. This is accomplished in a manner similar to that of assisting into P on E. The therapist straddles the patient's hips, and with MCs on the lateral clavicles assists the patient into the on-hands position.

If the patient is too large for the therapist to straddle, the therapist may have to stand lateral to the patient's hips with the patient's hips leaning against the therapist's legs (Fig. 30D). This is a somewhat less stable method but may be the only alternative.

When the quadruped position is achieved, approximation through the shoulders and the hips is applied. The therapist then moves to or stays at the side of the patient in preparation for the next procedure.

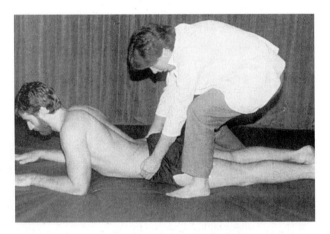

30A Quadruped: Initiation of movement.

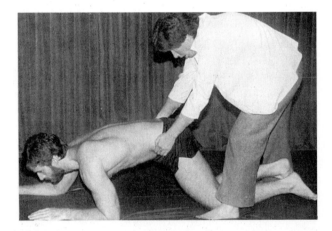

30B Quadruped: Midrange, patient walking back with the upper extremities.

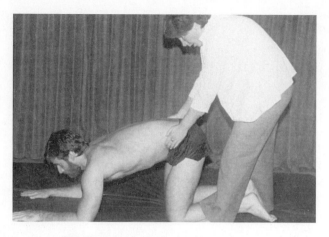

30C Quadruped: 90° flexion hips and knees.

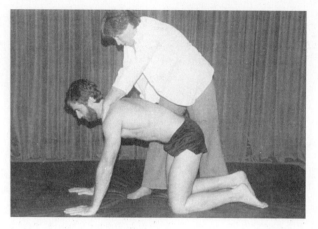

30D Quadruped: Completed range. Patient is assisted onto hands.

Purpose/Treatment Goals

The purpose is to assist a patient who cannot independently assume the position.

This procedure, as described, is most appropriate for SCI patients and will need to be modified for patients with other disabilities.

Problems with Application

The therapist may not walk back with the patient and therefore limit the patient's ability to flex the hips and the knees sufficiently to be stable in the position. Conversely, the therapist may pull the patient too far back into lower extremity flexion and heel sitting.

If the patient has excessive lower extremity extensor tone, the patient's feet can be positioned against a wall so that mass leg flexion can be more easily accomplished. Extensor tone may be decreased by preceding the activity with a quick movement into head flexion or increasing the amount of pelvic rotation.

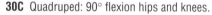

Activity: Quadruped

Technique: Rhythmic stabilization (RS); MC scapula; scapula and pelvis; pelvis

Impairments: Decreased postural stability in scapula, shoulder, upper or lower trunk or hips; decreased endurance of scapular, shoulder, upper or lower trunk or hip musculature.

31

Description

If the patient can maintain the quadruped position, AI may not be needed. The technique of RS can be applied to further enhance stability in the posture.

The therapist is positioned half-kneeling or standing near the patient's shoulders. To perform RS and provide resistance simultaneously in three directions, MCs are positioned on both scapulae. Similar to P on E, one MC resists in the rotational direction around C7 and the other resists in a diagonal direction. The heels of the therapist's hands are positioned below the spine of the scapula and the flat part of the fingers are around the top of the scapula (Fig. 31A). The resistive forces are smoothly altered without relaxation to promote simultaneous contraction around the weight-bearing segments.

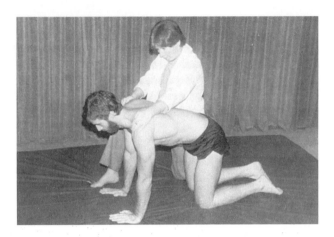

31A MC both scapulae emphasizing upper body stability.

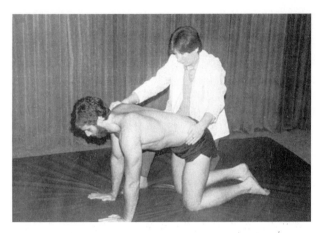

31B MC scapula and contralateral pelvis, emphasizing trunk stability.

To promote stability of the total trunk, MCs can be changed to one scapula and the opposite pelvis (Fig. 31B). Because there is no bony prominence on the dorsum of the pelvis, resistance to the pelvis is difficult to control and the hand will tend to slide. Rotational resistance is provided around the focal point of T12, the thoracolumbar junction. The hand on the pelvis applies primarily rotational resistance in the transverse plane and the contact on the scapula resists in the diagonal direction.

When both hands are placed on the pelvis, the focal point is lowered to the lumbar spine. As the placement of MCs is changed, the therapist's position also is altered to a more caudal position to assure a good biomechanical alignment from which to resist the diagonal direction (Fig. 31C).

Purpose/Treatment Goals

The purposes are to: (1) facilitate contraction of the total trunk musculature, (2) facilitate contraction of the upper extremity with the shoulder in 90 degrees of flexion and with more weight bearing than occurs in P on E, (3) enhance stability around an extended elbow, (4) promote contraction of the lower trunk and hip muscles, and (5) teach the patient with SCI to stabilize the lower trunk by controlling it through the upper body.

The therapist should be aware of the amount of arm participation when resistance is applied at the pelvis. MC on the pelvis can be used as an indirect approach to activate the upper extremity musculature.

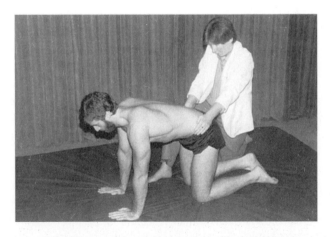

31C MCs on pelvis emphasizing lower trunk stability.

Problems with Application

The therapist may still have difficulty with the smooth transitions of isometric resistance required with RS. Resisting with each hand separately before putting the two resistive forces together may help to alleviate the problem. To promote the desired isometric control, care must be taken to gradually increase and decrease the resistance in each direction without allowing relaxation between contractions. The MC should be placed so that minimal or no movement occurs as the resistive forces are changed.

Frequently, therapists do not alter their position when different body parts are emphasized and consequently do not always apply resistance in the proper direction.

If the patient has difficulty performing simultaneous contractions and maintaining the lower trunk position, muscle stability in the shortened range of the extensors in pivot prone or a modified position may need to be emphasized.

	Mobility	Stability	Controlled Mobility	Skill
Quadruped	Assist to position	Rhythmic stabilization	Slow reversal hold	Resisted progression

Activity: Quadruped; diagonal rocking

Technique: Slow reversal hold (SRH) through increments of range; MC pelvis

Impairments: Decreased strength in trunk and extremities; decreased scapulohumeral dynamic stability at approximately 90 degrees of shoulder flexion; decreased stability in the elbow with increased body weight resistance; decreased dynamic control of lumbar and hip musculature.

Description

Weight shifting or rocking in weight-bearing positions promotes the controlled mobility stage of control. Rocking can be performed in the cephalocaudal, medial-lateral, and diagonal directions. Unless there is a specific reason to do each direction individually, rocking in a diagonal direction, which incorporates all motions, is preferred.

The therapist, in half-kneeling, is positioned near the patient's hips with MCs on the pelvis. The patient is directed to rock up and over the shoulder opposite to the therapist and back to the lower extremity nearer the therapist (Figs. 32A, 32B). The command may be "rock forward away from me and back toward me." The therapist applies a slight, quick stretch in the direction opposite to the desired movement. The resulting contraction is resisted through a small range. The command to "hold" is given at the end of that range and the isometric contraction is resisted. Quick stretch and resistance are applied to facilitate movement in the antagonistic direction followed by an isometric contraction. With each subsequent reversal, more range is allowed, i.e., moving through increments of range, until full range is achieved.

Purpose/Treatment Goals

The purposes are to enhance postural control responses; to develop the ability to independently assume the posture as increments of range are achieved; to promote controlled mobility; and, to

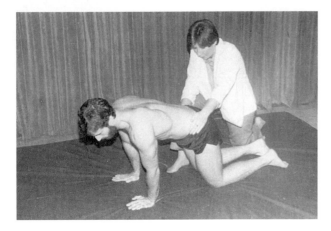

32A Rocking: Forward.

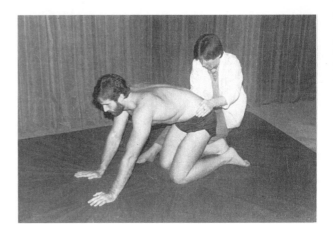

32B Rocking: Backward.

promote dynamic stability in the trunk and proximal muscles. Rocking from the midposition toward the heels can be used to promote trunk and extremity flexor tone and from midposition forward to promote extensor tone.

The proximal dynamic stability promoted in this procedure is appropriate for many patients including those with scapular or shoulder dysfunction. There is a difference in the motion performed and the amount of weight bearing between the two arms. The arm and leg toward which the patient is forwardly moving are in a D2 pattern and support more weight than the other limbs, which are moving in a D1 direction. For patients with shoulder dysfunction, the treatment plan usually emphasizes the D1 pattern before the D2. Therefore, weight bearing can be gradually increased with these patients by progressing the direction of rocking toward the uninvolved before the involved arm. The 90-degree range of shoulder flexion is problematic for many patients indicating a need for the development of dynamic stability in this range. If the patient cannot assume a quadruped position because of lower extremity or trunk limitations, the 90-degree position of the upper extremity can be achieved by upper extremity weight bearing against a wall while standing.

For patients with low back dysfunction the backward rocking motion may be indicated to enhance movement into hip flexion and to elongate low back extensors. Some patients with lumbar spine involvement are encouraged to maintain a relatively stable position in the lumbar spine avoiding excessive lumbar flexion or extension during the forward and backward rocking motion.

Knee flexion through full range occurs as backward rocking is increased; the pressure on the quadriceps tendon may diminish quadriceps responses.

This procedure does not effectively increase ROM although it is a good home exercise procedure to maintain the range gained during direct treatment. Sufficient ROM to maintain the position is a prerequisite. Mobility-ROM is first gained with mobilization and relaxation techniques. Weight shifting in quadruped enhances muscular control through the existing range.

Problems with Application

If the therapist is not diagonally posterior, the patient's movement will be difficult to control. Too vigorous a stretch may disturb the patient's balance and interfere with the smooth reversal of antagonists. If the scapula lifts of the thorax or excessively abducts, the procedure may be too difficult indicating the need for a less challenging procedure. For example, reducing upper extremity weight bearing by weight shifting in modified plantigrade (Procedure 62) or further promoting stability in quadruped.

Because of the amount of weight-bearing through the arm and the stress on the wrist and the hand, this position may not be appropriate for hemiplegics, except for those in the final stages of rehabilitation.

Patients with knee pain may find this weight-bearing position uncomfortable. A pillow under the knee may alleviate discomfort. The weight-bearing pressure and prolonged quadriceps stretch may diminish quadriceps strength counter to the goal for most patients with knee pathology during the early phases of rehabilitation.

Activity: Quadruped; weight shifting
Technique: Slow reversal hold (SRH) through decrements of range > AI > RS; MC pelvis
Impairments: Decreased postural stability; decreased ability to hold in mid range.

33

Description

The technique of rocking through decrements of range is appropriate for patients who cannot achieve the stability stage of motor control through the techniques of SHRC, AI, or RS. The patient with ataxia or athetosis may have uncontrolled movements with little or no ability to perform midline holding.

The therapist is positioned in the diagonal, posterior to the patient, with MCs on the pelvis or the pelvis and the shoulder. The large degree of movement through which the patient moves is gradually decreased until midline holding is accomplished. Holds are introduced first at the extremes of range and then through decrements of range until holding in the midline occurs. The technique then becomes AI and progresses to RS.

Purpose/Treatment Goals

The purpose is to enhance stability and midline holding in patients who cannot achieve stability in the more common fashion.

The technique of SRH through decrements of range is appropriately performed in the weight-bearing posture of quadruped where the approximation of body weight can assist the facilitation of midline holding or in other weight-bearing postures such as modified plantigrade or sitting.

The patient may need assistance with trunk support which can be provided by a bolster, ball, or stool.

Activity: Quadruped; D1, D2 UE; D1, D2 LE
Technique: Slow reversal hold (SRH); slow reversal (SR) or active movement; MC scapula (shoulder) and arm; thigh and foot
Impairments: Decreased dynamic stability in trunk and weight-bearing limbs; decreased controlled movement or strength in the trunk and proximal segments; decreased endurance in the trunk musculature.

34

Description

This procedure further promotes dynamic stability of the trunk and proximal musculature. To enhance upper body control, the upper extremity patterns are performed.

The therapist is in a half-kneeling position at the side of the patient. One MC is on the scapula (shoulder) of the weight-bearing arm to approximate and assist with balance. The other MC is on the forearm of the dynamic arm. The dynamic limb is guided first into the D1 pattern. The arm flexes across the face in D1F and extends toward the hip in D1E. The therapist is positioned on the diagonal so as not to interfere with the movement of the patient's arm (Figs. 34A, 34B). The dynamic limb also can be resisted in the D2 pattern. In D2F the thumb points toward the ceiling and in D2E toward the opposite knee (Figs. 34C, 34D). The amount of resistance applied to the uninvolved dynamic arm is dependent on the status of the involved static arm.

To perform the lower extremity patterns, the therapist moves caudally, remaining in a half-

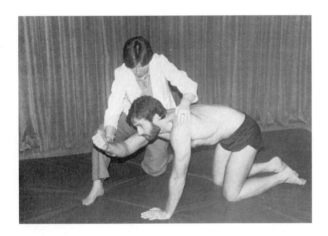

34A D1F, UE.

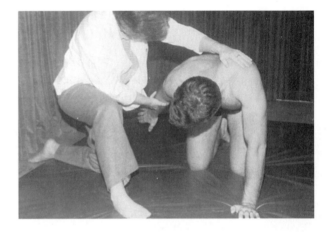

34B D1E, UE.

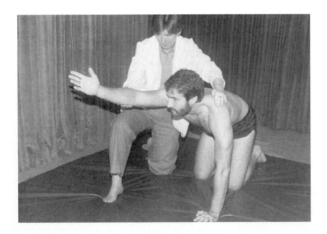

34C D2F, UE.

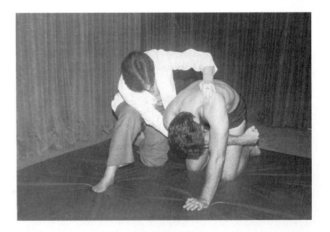

34D D2E, UE.

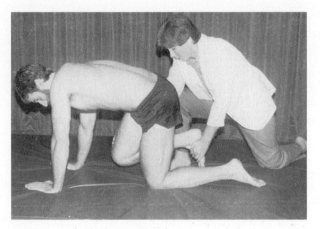

34E D1F, LE.

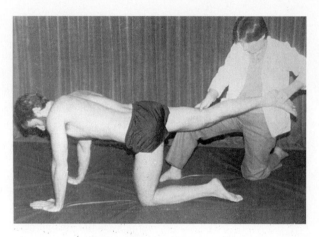

34F D1E, LE.

kneeling position. The lower extremity patterns are performed as mass flexion and extension motions. To resist the D1 flexor pattern, MCs are positioned on the anterior surface of the thigh and foot and the therapist instructs the patient to move the knee toward the opposite shoulder. During the D1 extensor pattern the leg extends and abducts toward the ceiling with resistance provided by MCs on the posterior thigh and plantar surface of the foot (Figs. 34E, 34F). The D2 pattern of the LE combines hip flexion with abduction and hip extension with adduction. Enhancing the proximal component of the D2 pattern is not commonly needed and is not usually performed in quadruped. Contralateral limbs can be lifted simultaneously to further improve control of the back extensors. Dynamic postural control is challenged with these movements (Procedure 145).

The challenge of the procedures increases as the dynamic limb(s) moves through greater excursions of range and as resistive forces increase. Trunk and proximal stability can be enhanced as the dynamic limbs hold in shortened ranges of shoulder flexion and lower extremity extension; more dynamic proximal stability is challenged if the limbs rhythmically move apart and together.

Purpose/Treatment Goals

The purposes are: to improve the dynamic stability of the muscles around the weight-bearing joints and the static limbs; to enhance the strength of the dynamic limb; to promote movement in the thoracic spine; to emphasize lumbar movement and pelvic rotation; and to promote balance and coordination.

These static–dynamic activities are effective as part of a home program for patients with scoliosis and shoulder, thoracic, lumbar or hip involvement. The upper limb D2 pattern combines trunk flexion or extension with rotation; the D1 pattern promotes lateral trunk flexion or elongation. When performing the arm patterns, the lumbar spine is relatively stable by virtue of weight bearing and movement occurs primarily in the thoracic region. When the lower extremity patterns are performed, the trunk movement occurs primarily in the lumbar spine.

For patients with shoulder dysfunction, increased dynamic stability occurs as the uninvolved limb is lifted off the surface. The appropriateness of inclusion in the treatment plan is determined by the ability to dynamically stabilize the scapula without "winging," or excessive abduction or muscle flickering indicating fatigue.

For patients with thoracic involvement, thoracic extension is enhanced with shoulder flexion movements, primarily D2F, and thoracic flexion is promoted with shoulder extension, particularly D2E.

For those with lumbar involvement, low back and hip extension is promoted with D1E. This motion challenges dynamic stability in the lumbar region. Residual tightness of hip flexors and weakness of the abdominals may result in excessive lumbar extension. These muscle impairments may need to be corrected before full range of lower extremity motion is appropriate. Conversely, during the hip flexion motion excessive lumbar flexion may occur if the lumbar extensors do not adequately respond or if range into hip flexion is limited.

If the patient has good upper extremity control, the quadruped position can be used effectively to improve hip or LE function. In this position gravity and tone assist the flexor movement, therefore the therapist can provide increased manual resistance. The movement into mass flexion may enhance overflow from stronger to weaker segments. Hip extension is resisted by gravity and tonal influences. Manual resistance or weights can further challenge the response. The technique of repeated contractions (RC) can be added to the extensor motions to emphasize the hip extension component of the pattern.

Problems with Application

When performing the upper extremity patterns the therapist may position the MC too distally on the dynamic limb. The MC should be positioned more proximally near the elbow to control the full excursion of movement. Because the primary purpose of these static–dynamic procedures is to improve control in the trunk and weight-bearing limbs, specific distal movements need not be emphasized. When performing the leg pattern the therapist should be in a half-kneeling position far enough posterior to the patient to provide adequate resistance through the entire range. Cuff weights and elastic bands can be used to provide resistance as part of an independent or home program.

35

Activity: Side sitting to quadruped

Technique: Guided transitional movement; MC pelvis or scapula and pelvis

Impairments: Decreased pelvic rotational control; decreased ability to shift weight.

Description

The transition from side sitting to quadruped is an example of the many transitional movements that can be performed. The patient is in a side sitting position and the therapist is positioned behind the patient with MCs on the pelvis. The pelvis is guided laterally until the quadruped position is reached. To discourage abnormal movement, rotation of the trunk is facilitated. From the quadruped position the patient can be returned to side sitting on the same or opposite side. Because the goal is independent movement, as little assistance as possible is provided in this procedure.

Purpose/Treatment Goals

The purposes are: to facilitate the ability to move from one posture to another; to promote normal automatic righting and postural responses needed during transitional movements; and to promote proximal dynamic control.

Problems with Application

Patients are ready for this type of activity only after developing stability and controlled mobility in the posture. Therapists may attempt transitional movements before these prerequisite stages of movement control are enhanced.

Activity: Creeping
Technique: Resisted progression (RP); MC ankles or pelvis
Impairments: Poor control of lumbar, pelvic, and hip regions during skilled movement; poor proximal dynamic stability.

36

Description

Locomotion in the quadruped position or creeping is the skill level of control in this posture. A developmental progression exists within the locomotive pattern. Bunny hopping combines a symmetrical pattern of extremity movement and flexion-extension movements of the trunk. An ipsilateral pattern combines extremity movements on the same side of the body with lateral trunk bending. The most advanced pattern first combines sequential and then simultaneous contralateral motions of the extremities with trunk counterrotation.

To emphasize the lower extremity movement the therapist is positioned behind the patient with MCs on the ankles. The patient shifts weight onto one lower extremity. A stretch is given to the flexor motion of the unweighted leg (Fig. 36A) and tracking resistance is provided until the knee is in a position to bear weight (Fig. 36B). Weight is shifted onto that leg and the other leg is stretched and resisted. The patient controls the movement of the upper extremities independently or on the cue of verbal commands.

The progression of motion can be in a straight or a diagonal direction. With a diagonal progression the ipsilateral extremities leading the movement are in the D2 pattern and the other extremities move in D1. When facilitating extension or creeping backward, the MCs are positioned on the ankles or soles of the feet. A stretch to the extensor pattern of one leg is followed by tracking resistance.

To facilitate rotation and protraction of the pelvis, MCs can also be positioned on the pelvis

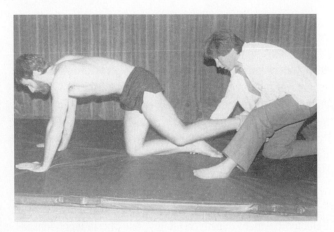

36A Stretch in mid range to flexor movement.

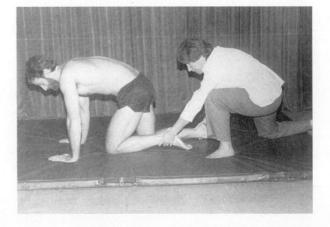

36B Weight bearing on support limbs.

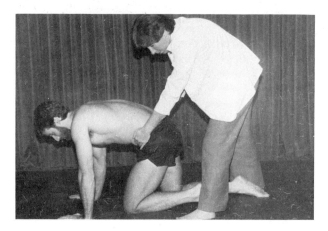

36C Guiding movement at trunk.

during forward locomotion (Fig. 36C). The stretch to the pelvis is applied in an upward elongation motion to encourage protraction and rotation of the pelvis as the leg moves into flexion. The posterior motion with MCs on the pelvis is not usually performed.

Purpose/Treatment Goals

The purpose of this procedure is to enhance the locomotive pattern by promoting the combination of extremity and trunk motions as well as enhancing skilled movements, especially in the leg. Creeping in a forward direction promotes lower trunk and extremity flexion and creeping in a backward direction promotes lower trunk and extremity extension. These procedures may be useful for children with diminished lumbar, pelvic, and hip control or with adults with incomplete spinal cord involvement or those with generalized weakness such as Guillian–Barré or multiple sclerosis.

Problems with Application

The patient may attempt to move too quickly and the therapist may lose control of the movements. When performed in a slow, deliberate fashion, the correct movement patterns can be enhanced.

Summary

We have completed the activities in the prone sequence emphasizing pivot prone and the weight-bearing postures of prone on elbows and quadruped. In each of these positions we began by assisting the patient to the position, the mobility stage of movement control. The patient must have the ROM to assume the posture and must be able to initiate the movement. An increase in abnormal tone, which occurs at attempts to attain or maintain the position, is usually indicative of too much stress. If this occurs, a less stressful posture should be used. Muscle stability was promoted in pivot prone as the position was maintained. Postural stability, or the ability to maintain the position, was developed in the weight-bearing postures with the techniques of AI and RS. Controlled mobility, weight shifting, was promoted with the technique of SRH through increments of range to enhance balance, dynamic stability, and the independent assumption of the posture. Static–dynamic activities promoted with SR, SRH, RC, and active movement emphasized control in the trunk and weight-bearing limbs. Skill was gained in quadruped by applying RP to a reciprocal creeping pattern.

Lower Trunk Progression

ACTIVITIES

Lower trunk rotation
Bridging
Kneeling
Half kneeling

FACTORS RELATING TO THE PROGRESSION OF ACTIVITIES

Biomechanical Factors

Base of support decreases
Center of gravity (mass) elevates from surface
Resistance
   Elongated lever arm in lower extremities
   Manual contacts proximal to distal
   Effects of gravity and weight bearing increased

Reflexive Factors

Increased tonic influences in supine
Decreased tonic influences in kneeling
Increased righting reactions in kneeling
Increased need for postural control in hooklying and kneeling

	Mobility	Stability	Controlled Mobility	Skill
Lower trunk rotation	Rhythmic initiation	Alternating isometrics	Slow reversal hold	
	Hold relax active motion	Rhythmic stabilization		

Activity: Lower trunk rotation (LTR)

Technique: Rhythmic initiation (RI); MC knees

Impairments: Decreased ROM in the lower trunk associated with hypertonia, rigidity, pain and stiffness in lumbar joints and muscles; decreased ability to initiate active movement.

37

Description

The patient is positioned in hooklying. The therapist is at the patient's side with MCs on the knees. Most of the procedures performed in this position involve rotational movements that can be controlled better from this lateral position with the therapist in line with the movement.

As previously mentioned, the technique of RI begins with passive movement. In hooklying, rotation of the lower trunk occurs when the knees are moved laterally in both directions (Figs. 37A, 37B). As the patient relaxes, the ROM is gradually increased. The amount of patient effort also can be increased from passive, through active assistive, to tracking resistance. During the passive and assistive phases, MCs are on both sides of the knees to assist the movement. In the

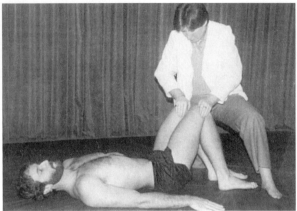

37A RI: LTR

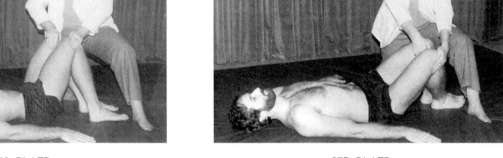

37B RI: LTR

tracking resistive phase, MCs are in the direction of the patient's movement. If the patient is not hyperreflexive a slight stretch can be applied in the lengthened range of the pattern to facilitate the isotonic movement. To reiterate, RI begins with passive movements through small ranges, then the range, amount of patient effort and speed of the movement are increased gradually.

Purpose/Treatment Goals

The purposes are to promote rotational motion in the lower trunk, crossing of the midline, the interaction of the two sides of the body and the reversal of antagonists; to reduce muscle and joint stiffness, and to enhance relaxation.

The activity includes flexor and extensor phases. The motion that occurs from the lengthened range to midposition is the flexor phase, i.e., it facilitates and is performed by trunk and hip flexors; motion from the mid- to shortened position is the extensor phase, that facilitates lower trunk and hip extensors.

RI is appropriate to gain mobility primarily in patients with hypertonia but can be useful to achieve relaxation for any patient with low back or hip tightness. If the patient is hemiparetic, the upper extremity may be positioned in shoulder extension with abduction, forearm supination, and wrist and finger extension to discourage synergistic patterns. The effort put forth by the patient is kept below a level that produces an associated reaction that interferes with function.

If specific pelvic motion rather than the combined pelvic and hip motion is desired, the therapist can place MCs directly on the pelvis. Conversely, hip motions and elongation of the tensor fascia lata can be encouraged by stabilizing the pelvis with one MC and promoting hip motion with the other contact on the knees.

Problems with Application

Therapists may inappropriately position themselves at the patient's feet rather than at the side. Such positioning prevents the therapist from using body mechanics effectively for the application of assistance or resistance.

The procedure is intended to promote rotational motion in the lower and not in the entire trunk. Total trunk movement can be the result of muscular or joint tightness, hypertonia, or splinting due to pain. If total body motion occurs, the therapist should reduce the range of movement until the motion is isolated to the lower trunk area. MC on the thorax may discourage this tendency.

Because of abnormal tone or a hyperactive positive support reflex, the patient's feet may tend to slide away from the buttocks. This tendency can be reduced by blocking the patient's feet with the therapist's foot. When blocking the feet, however, the therapist may incorrectly bear weight on the dorsum of the patient's foot, thereby limiting inversion and eversion. In addition, this excessive pressure on the soles of the feet may increase the tendency toward mass extension. A better alternative may be to direct weight-bearing pressure onto the heels with a wedge or support placed under the soles of the feet. This alteration of foot pressure may be necessary for all of the procedures performed in the hooklying and bridging positions.

Activity: Lower trunk rotation (LTR)

Techniques: Hold relax active motion (HRAM); MC knees

Impairments: Decreased strength lower trunk and hip musculature (1-2/5); asymmetry of lower extremity strength.

38

Description

This procedure promotes the mobility stage of motor control, the ability to initiate movement. The therapist is lateral to the patient and is on the side opposite the direction of movement to be emphasized. Before the technique is applied the patient is passively moved through the range of lower trunk rotation to assess flexibility. The need for this technique is determined by applying a quick stretch in the lengthened range of the movement. If the patient has difficulty initiating the movement or sustaining the contraction throughout the range, the muscles may lack sufficient actin-myosin bonding, stretch sensitivity, or alpha-gamma coactivation to initiate or sustain the contraction.

With the weakened muscles in their shortened range, the technique begins with an isometric contraction resisted for a few seconds (Fig. 38A). After relaxing the isometric contraction in the shortened range, the legs are passively and quickly moved into the lengthened range (Fig. 38B). A quick stretch is applied and the subsequent isotonic contraction is resisted back into the shortened range. During the initial portion of the movement, with the legs moving against gravity, manual assistance may be needed. Verbal commands should accompany each phase of the technique: "hold," during the isometric contraction in the shortened range; "relax," while the legs are passively moved by the therapist into the lengthened range; "now move your legs

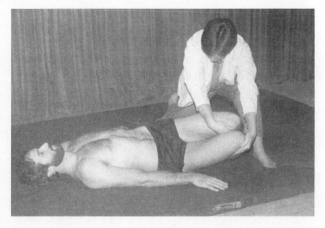

38A HRAM to LTR: Holding shortened range.

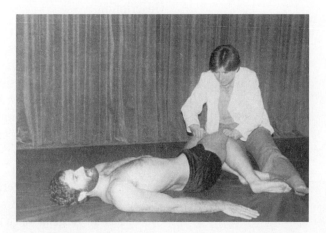

38B HRAM to LTR: Quick stretch in lengthened range.

away from me," as the quick stretch is applied and the resulting movement is resisted or assisted into the shortened range. Minimal tracking resistance is applied throughout the motion to facilitate the contraction. Increased resistance can be applied as the response improves.

Purpose/Treatment Goals

The purpose is to promote the initiation of active motion, the mobility stage of control, for patients with weakness or hypotonia, e.g., Guillian–Barré syndrome or muscular dystrophy.

The goals are for the patient to initiate the movement and move with increased strength throughout range. The resisted isometric contraction is performed to recruit gamma motor neurons and to develop muscle spindle stretch sensitivity. If this occurs, the patient may better respond to the stretch applied in the lengthened range. In addition to altering spindle sensitivity, the isometric contraction may enhance actin-myosin bonding to facilitate subsequent contractions in lengthened ranges.

Problems with Application

Therapists often begin the passive movement into the lengthened range before the patient has completely relaxed the isometric contraction. Although the legs must be quickly returned to the lengthened range after the hold, enough time must be allowed so the patient can relax.

The stretch in the lengthened range must be coordinated with the verbal command to "move your legs away." Such summation of sensory inputs may enhance the patient's response.

The range of the movement may vary with each patient. The patient may have been on bed rest or may have some natural tightness. Overstretching should be avoided with this procedure. If ROM needs to be increased, other techniques such as HR or RI can be applied (Procedure 37).

39

Activity: Hooklying

Technique: Alternating isometrics (AI) progressing to rhythmic stabilization (RS) (AI > RS); MC knees, ankles

Impairments: Decreased strength lower abdominals; poor lower trunk stability; decreased stability of the hip and knee musculature in mid ranges.

Description

The techniques of AI and RS applied in hooklying develop stability in the lower trunk and hip musculature with the extensors of the hip and the knee on stretch. The therapist is positioned on a diagnonal near the patient's feet in line with the lower abdominals. With MCs positioned on the knees, AI is performed with resistance applied in a diagonal direction away from and toward the therapist (Figs. 39A, 39B). With AI, muscle activity is alternately produced in the abdominals and the back extensors. RS is performed to facilitate contraction on both sides of the segments simultaneously. To achieve RS, resistance is simultaneously applied in alternate directions with both MCs, one knee is pushed away as the other is pulled toward the therapist (Fig. 39C).

These two techniques can also be applied with MCs on the ankles to increase the activation of the hip and knee musculature. With AI, both MCs pull toward or away from the therapist (Figs. 39D, 39E). In RS, the MCs resist in opposite directions.

To alter the range in which the muscles are being activated, the legs can be placed in more extension (Fig. 39F). The lower extremities can also be separated, which may increase the activation of the hip muscles; either limb may be facilitated unilaterally (Fig. 39G).

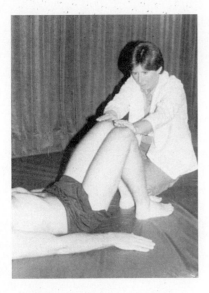

39A AI: Resistance to extension.

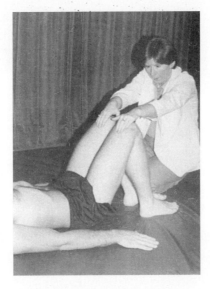

39B AI: Resistance to flexion.

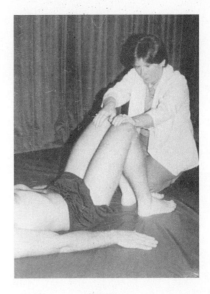

39C RS.

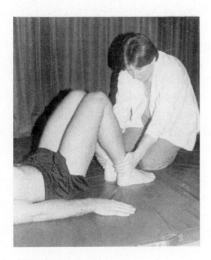

39D AI: Resistance to flexion.

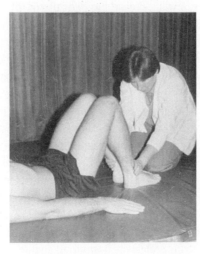

39E AI: Resistance to extension.

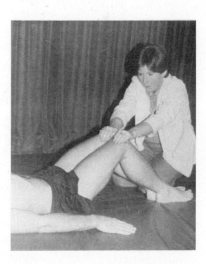

39F Decreasing hip and knee flexion angle.

Purpose/Treatment Goals

The purpose is to enhance alternating or simultaneous isometric contractions of the trunk, hip, and knee musculature.

This procedure is appropriate for most patients with low back dysfunction. The hooklying position minimizes the pressure within the disc, the compressive forces on the lumbar facets and the need for postural stability. The stability techniques of AI and RS can focus on improving muscle stability without the need to maintain a weight-bearing posture. Regardless of the specific diagnosis increasing endurance or strengthening of the lower trunk muscles, especially the lower abdominals, is usually indicated. Low intensity isometric contractions can be performed early in treatment because they cause minimal, if any, discomfort, and a normal breathing pattern can be maintained. To challenge the abdominals more and to simulate the upright position, the legs are moved into more extension and the techniques reapplied. MCs positioned on the

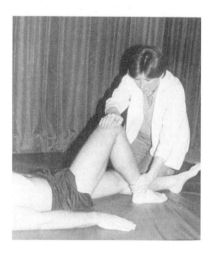

39G Unilateral hip and knee flexion.

ankles will increase the length of the lever arm. The increased extension and the distal placement of the MCs will increase the difficulty of the procedure by progressively increasing the stress or resistance to the lower abdominals.

Hemiplegic patients and others with increased extensor tone in the lower limbs also may benefit from these procedures by promoting a balance of tone in the lower extremity musculature. This may be achieved by activation of the hamstring muscles followed by a slowly graded contraction of the quadriceps without eliciting a spastic response. This rhythmic reversal of antagonist contractions and smooth muscle reversals is needed during ambulation. Patients with hypertonia have difficulty gradually increasing then releasing or relaxing the contraction of the spastic muscle and subsequently activating the antagonist. This procedure is designed to help alleviate these problems. For hemiplegic patients the progression would be from a trunk or bilateral posture to a unilateral holding of the hemiplegic limb with the hip and knee in decreasing amounts of flexion. The speed of the contractions and the amount of isometric resistance is gradually increased.

Stability around the knee can be promoted with the knee in various ranges. If, for example, improved hamstring stability is desired, AI and RS can be promoted with the knee progressively in more extension.

Stability may be developed more easily in hooklying as compared to quadruped and sitting because less weight bearing occurs in this posture with less stretch on the extensors. Hooklying, however, a supine position, may be more difficult if the patient has increased extensor tone or an exaggerated positive support reflex.

Problems with Application

The therapist incorrectly may be positioned in front of the patient rather than in a diagonal direction. If resistance is applied in this straight plane the muscle activated may be primarily the rectus abdominus, which is the less postural portion of the abdominals. The resistance applied at the knees should attempt to flex or extend the hips and the knees in a diagonal direction.

When MCs are placed on the ankles to facilitate hip and knee extension, resistance is directed backward toward the buttocks and not down into the heels.

Summary

This procedure can be progressed by altering the (1) activity: positioning the legs in more extension, separating the legs or performing unilaterally, and the (2) technique: AI to RS with increasing speed and resistance and positioning the MCs from the knees to the ankles.

Activity: Lower trunk rotation (LTR)
Technique: Slow reversal hold (SRH) with repeated contractions (RC); MC knees
Impairments: Decreased trunk rotation; decreased interaction of body sides; weakness of proximal musculature.

40

Description

This procedure is designed to enhance a controlled contraction of trunk and hip musculature in the direction of trunk rotation. The therapist is in a half-kneeling position at the patient's side opposite the side of weakness. The patient is passively moved through the range a few times to determine the existing range and to teach the patient the movement. SRH begins in the lengthened range with a quick stretch (Fig. 40A). The isotonic contraction is resisted throughout the available range followed by an isometric contraction at the end of range (Fig. 40B). The antagonistic motion is facilitated with a quick stretch and the reversal motion resisted in the same manner (Figs. 40C, 40D). This reversal of movements is continued in a smooth fashion without relaxation or loss of the contraction. Resistance should be increased with each reversal whenever possible. One MC can be placed on the pelvis to emphasize forward rotation of the lower trunk (Fig. 40E).

    The technique of repeated contractions (RC) may be added if weakness is present in any part of the range. RC may enhance the strength of the contraction by superimposing quick stretches on the isotonic contraction. If weakness is most evident in the beginning of the range or the patient has difficulty initiating movement, repeated stretches can be applied in the lengthened range to facilitate the contraction. If weakness is present throughout the range, the quick stretches can be superimposed throughout the isotonic movement wherever the weakness is felt. When weakness is primarily in the shortened range, most commonly in extensors, the pat-

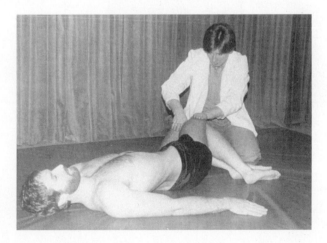

40A LTR: Quick stretch in lengthened range.

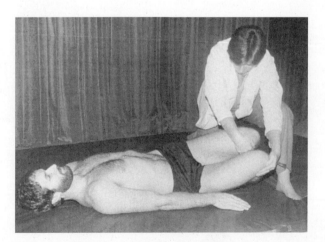

40B LTR: Hold in the shortened range.

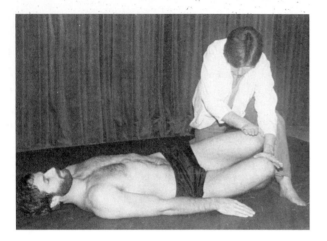

40C LTR: Quick stretch to the antagonist.

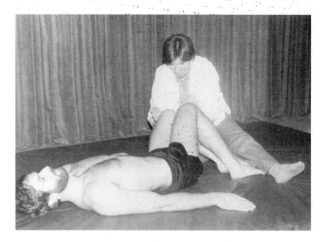

40D LTR: Hold to the antagonist in shortened range.

tern is resisted to the point of weakness and an isometric contraction performed to further enhance muscle spindle activity at that point. This is followed by RC into the remaining range.

Purpose/Treatment Goals

The activity of LTR will promote rotation in the lower trunk, crossing of the midline, and an interaction of flexor and extensor muscles. The technique of SRH will promote strengthening and a smooth reversal of antagonists. The technique of RC is used to enhance the strength of the contraction either at the initiation of the movement, throughout the range or in the shortened range. With RC the summation of the voluntary and the reflex contraction should facilitate more motor unit firing.

For patients with disc pathology, the range of lower trunk rotation must be carefully monitored. Although small movements at midrange may be within the patient's tolerance any large excursion of rotational movement may not be indicated.

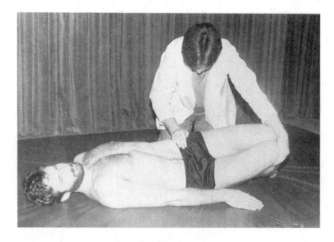

40E MC on knee and pelvis.

Problems with Application

Strong and specific verbal commands are necessary with RC. Frequently the patient will relax or move in the direction of the stretch. To enhance the patient's response, the manual stretch must be superimposed on an active muscle contraction. The amount of resistance applied to the contraction following the stretch must be carefully graded. Too little resistance will not sustain the muscle contraction and too much resistance will overcome the muscle response. The therapist must learn to apply resistance to sustain but not defeat the contraction.

Activity: Bridging

Technique: Alternating isometrics (AI) progressing to rhythmic stabilization (RS) (AI > RS); MC pelvis

Impairments: Decreased stability and strength in the lower trunk, hips, knees, and ankles; decreased ability to simultaneously contract the gluteus medius and maximus; decreased strength of hamstrings; dominance of abnormal synergistic patterns in the lower extremity.

41

Description

When the hips begin to extend off the supporting surface during the performance of an isometric contraction in the shortened range of LTR, the patient may be ready to progress to bridging. The patient may need assistance into the posture, but maintenance of the position should be independent before techniques are applied.

The therapist is positioned to the side of the patient's hips. With MCs on the pelvis, stability in bridging is first enhanced with the technique of AI. Resistance can be applied in the anterior-posterior (A-P) direction with MCs sliding from the anterior to the posterior pelvic region to facilitate primarily the low back and hip extensors (Figs. 41A, 41B). With MCs positioned on the lateral surface of the pelvis, AI can be applied in a medial-lateral (M-L) direction to facilitate the abdominals, the hip abductors, and adductors (Figs. 41C, 41D). AI to rotational movements of the pelvis will alternately enhance most of the trunk and hip muscles. The rotational resistance is applied in the transverse plane with one MC on the anterior surface rotating downward while the other MC is on the posterior pelvis rotating upward (Fig. 41E). To alter resistance, the MCs slide from one surface to the other without allowing relaxation between contractions.

RS applied to the pelvis in bridging combines resistance in a diagonal and rotational direction

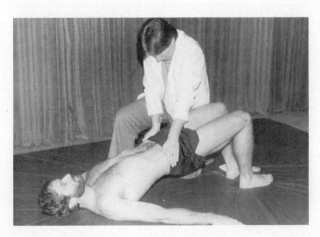

41A AI: Resistance to trunk extension.

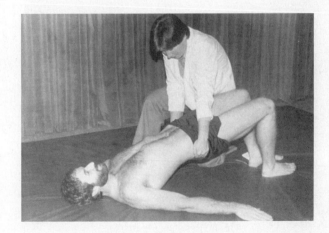

41B AI: Resistance to flexion.

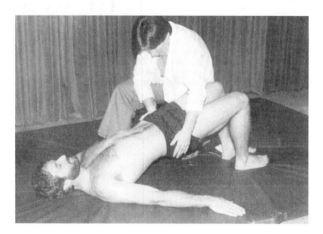

41C AI: Resistance to medial lateral direction.

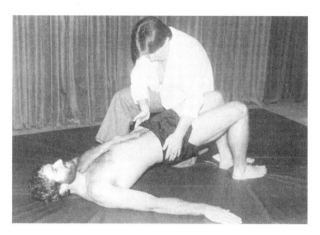

41D AI: Resistance to medial lateral direction.

and enhances simultaneous contraction of the lower trunk and hip muscles. One MC provides resistance primarily in the diagonal direction and the other MC primarily to rotation (Fig. 41F).

With the knee flexed, the hamstrings are in a position of active insufficiency and hip extension is performed primarily with the gluteus maximus. The range of knee extension can be increased, which will increase activity of the hamstrings. The challenge to the lower body can be increased and dynamic stability promoted by positioning a ball under the thighs, legs, or feet. The upper extremities can be lifted from the surface or the upper body positioned on a ball, which will decrease the stability provided by the upper body.

Purpose/Treatment Goals

The purposes are to (1) enhance lower trunk and hip stability in the shortened ranges of these muscles, (2) promote advanced patterns of the lower extremity, i.e., hip extension and knee flexion, (3) challenge the patient to maintain knee flexion in the supine position, (4) promote simultaneous contractions of the gluteus maximus and gluteus medius, and (5) enhance activity of the hamstrings as the range of knee extension increases.

The patient maintains knee flexion in the supine position which requires that the influence of the symmetrical tonic labyrinthine reflex does not dominate motor behavior. As the patient maintains the lower trunk and hip position there is a simultaneous contraction of the gluteus max-

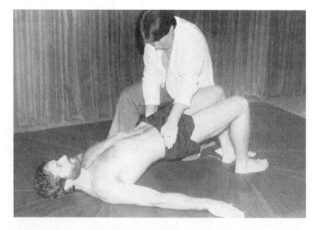

41E AI: Resistance to rotation.

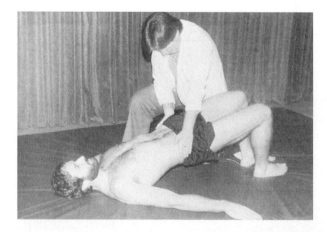

41F RS: Resistance in all three directions.

imus and medius in preparation for the stance phase of gait. Manual contacts can be positioned on the knees to increase resistance to abduction or an elastic band can be used for a home program.

Problems with Application

The therapist may be incorrectly positioned at the patient's feet resulting in poor use of body mechanics. When correctly positioned at the patient's side, the therapist can use upper body weight to apply resistance. Smooth transitions of MCs and of resistance may be difficult if the patient has a large pelvis, especially during resistance of rotational movements.

During AI to the pelvis in the A-P direction, the anterior or ventrally directed resistance ("don't let me lift you") is difficult for the therapist to apply in bridging. Resistance to flexor muscles can be more easily accomplished in other positions such as quadruped (Procedure 31).

If strength in the low back and hip extensors is deficient, a return to other less stressful activities, such as lower trunk extension, may be necessary to enhance muscle stability of the extensors. This can be accomplished by positioning the legs in the shortened range of extension and applying isometric resistance with approximation to the extensors to facilitate the holding contraction. The patient can practice muscle stability exercises independently by putting a pillow under the knees and performing a quadriceps and a gluteal set. Once the patient can sustainthis SRHC, the muscles may be better able to cope with the resistance of body weight in the bridging position.

	Mobility	Stability	Controlled Mobility	Skill
Bridging		Alternating isometrics Rhythmic stabilization	Slow reversal hold Agonistic reversals	Active movement

Activity: Bridging; pelvic motions, A-P, M-L, and rotation
Technique: Slow reversal hold (SRH): MC pelvis
Impairments: Decreased dynamic balance in the lower body; decreased ability to bear weight on one lower extremity; weakness in the gluteus maximus and medius; decreased time in unilateral stance.

42

Description

Once postural stability is established in bridging, weight shifting or controlled mobility can be promoted in the three planes of movement. With the therapist at the patient's side, MCs are placed on the anterior pelvis and the patient is instructed to elevate the hips from hooklying into the bridging position. Resistance is applied and a hold emphasized in the shortened range of lower trunk and hip extension. MCs are then changed to the posterior pelvis and resistance applied to the antagonistic motion or lowering of the hips to the mat. As previously mentioned, this lowering, a flexor motion, is difficult for the therapist to resist as the patient is assisted by gravity and thus is not emphasized. To perform SRH to pelvic rotation, one MC is placed on the anterior pelvis and the other on the posterior side of the other pelvis. A quick stretch is applied followed by resistance to the rotational motion and a hold in the shortened range. MCs are then altered to the opposite side of the pelvis and rotation resisted in the other direction (Fig. 42A). Emphasis is always placed on forward pelvic rotation with the commands "rotate your left hip forward, then rotate your right hip forward." SRH in the M-L direction is accomplished by placing MCs on alternate lateral sides of the pelvis (Fig. 42B). If the focus of the procedure is to improve the patient's ability to laterally shift during gait, the therapist must limit the lateral motion to the pelvis and the hips and prevent excessive lateral movement of the knees and the ankles.

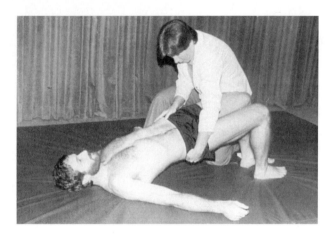

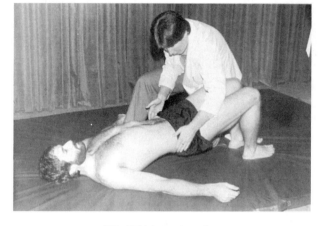

42A SRH: Rotational motion.   **42B** SRH: Lateral motion.

If, however, this procedure is being performed to improve motion at the ankles, lateral movements of the entire body may be desirable.

Purpose/Treatment Goals

The purposes are: (1) to enhance controlled movement in the posture, (2) to improve the pelvic determinants of gait, (3) to increase dynamic strength of the lower trunk extensors, and (4) to increase weight bearing on a lower extremity.

Pelvic movements are performed individually before they are combined into one smooth motion. Combined motions can be performed in bridging as well as in upright postures such as modified plantigrade and standing in stride.

The knees can be positioned together to increase sensory feedback or apart to increase the BoS depending on the patient's needs.

If these procedures are performed on a hemiplegic patient, the position of the UE is monitored to discourage associated reactions.

For patients with low back dysfunction, the lateral motion may be emphasized before promoting rotational movements.

Problems with Application

During the rotational movements the entire pelvis should stay in an elevated position and not drop or flex. To promote the control needed in gait, the lower trunk and hips should remain extended during the entire sequence.

When resistance is applied in the A-P and rotational directions, the therapist should slide, not lift, MCs from one surface to the other.

43

Activity: Bridging; pelvic elevation

Technique: Agonistic reversals (AR); MC pelvis

Impairments: Poor eccentric control in lumbar and hip extensors and hamstrings; decreased ability to control motion from standing to sitting.

Description

As stated, the major muscle groups activated in bridging are the low back and hip extensors. To enhance eccentric control of the extensor groups, the technique of AR is performed. With this technique there is an alteration of concentric–eccentric contractions of the extensors. The thera-

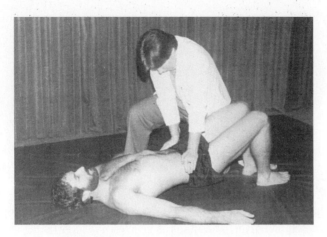

43A AR: Eccentric contraction of extensors.

pist places MCs on the anterior surface of the pelvis and resists the concentric extensor contraction as the patient elevates the pelvis. With MCs maintained on the anterior surface, an eccentric lowering of the pelvis is resisted combined with the verbal command of "make me work at pushing you down" or "lower yourself toward the mat slowly." The patient lowers the pelvis through a small range, eccentric concentration (Fig. 43A), then concentrically contracts at the command "now lift up your hips." This technique is usually performed through increments of range allowing the patient to move through more range, closer to the mat, with each reversal of concentric–eccentric contractions. An isometric contraction of the extensors in the shortened range may be performed to improve the subsequent eccentric control.

Purpose/Treatment Goals

The purpose is to enhance eccentric control of the low back and hip extensors. This is particularly appropriate for patients who have difficulty lowering themselves with control from a standing to a sitting position.

For patients with low back dysfunction, eccentric control of the low back and hip extensors is important. In bridging where there may be less joint and muscular strain, eccentric control may be less difficult to control compared with upright postures. Eccentric control through increments of range is particularly important for patients with increased tone in the extensors. The patient learns to control the gradual lengthening of the active muscle contraction. Eccentric control of the hamstrings can be promoted with the knees in greater amounts of extension. This simulates the range in which eccentric control is needed during ambulation.

Problems with Application

Instead of resisting an eccentric contraction, a therapist may incorrectly ask for an isometric contraction and increase resistance until the patient loses control. Carefully applied resistance combined with correct verbal commands ensure the proper sequence of contractions. Because extensor muscles seem to be inhibited as the lengthened range is reached, the technique is applied through increments of range.

44

Activity: Bridging; advanced treatment procedures

Technique: AI > RS > SRH, active motion; MC knees, ankles

Impairments: Decreased gluteus maximus and medius and hamstring strength and decreased control of ankle musculature; decreased ability to quickly initiate and alternate responses; decreased control of the stance phase of gait; decreased dynamic stability in the lower body.

Description

This sequence of exercises, usually performed toward the conclusion of the rehabilitation process, may be appropriate for patients who are returning to advanced functional levels. As in other procedures, each unit of the procedure can be altered to increase the difficulty or change the focus of the procedure.

To change the activity, the BoS can be altered by moving the feet further from the buttocks, which increases the activity of the hamstring muscles (Fig. 44A); the patient can perform unilateral weight-bearing (static–dynamic) activities, which increases the activation of all the muscles (Fig. 44B).

The techniques can be progressed from those promoting stability, AI and RS, to SRH and AR, which will enhance controlled mobility. Muscular contraction can also be progressed to fast alternating movements by having the patient first walk and then run in place in the bridging position. These quick movements can be combined with changing the knee angle into more extension. By having the patient move laterally during the running motions, the lateral ligaments can be stressed in this controlled condition.

The placement of MCs can begin on the pelvis, move to the knees, and then to the ankles (Figs. 44C, 44D), which increases the lever arm and the amount of muscle activity. During the fast alternate motions MCs are removed and the patient performs the procedure without the facilitation of this sensory input. The progression of these units within this procedure can all overlap.

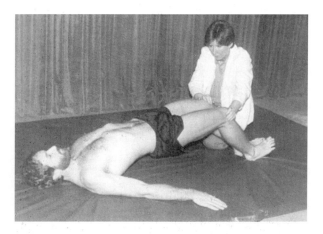

44A Knees in more extension MC on knees.

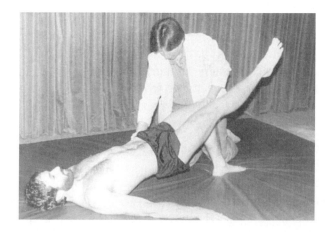

44B Unilateral weight-bearing MC pelvis and knee.

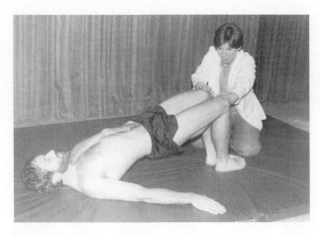

44C MC knees.

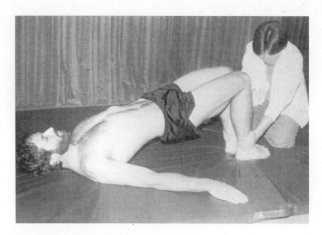

44D MC ankles.

Purpose/Treatment Goals

The purposes are: to supplement advanced gait training activities by emphasizing unilateral weight bearing; to enhance pelvic, knee, and ankle stability and simultaneous activation of the gluteus maximus and gluteus medius; to improve hamstring muscle control; to promote the dynamic stability needed for ambulation; and to promote fast bursts of muscular activity for patients returning to athletic events.

Problems with Application

Therapists may apply too much resistance with the distal placement of MCs, especially when the patient is unilaterally weight bearing. Maintenance of the position may provide enough stress for some patients. With the knee in full flexion, the hamstrings are in a position of active insufficiency, therefore, excessive resistance in this position directed toward the knee flexors may cause cramping.

Activity: Kneeling

Technique: Alternating isometrics progressing to rhythmic stabilization progressing to slow reversal hold (AI > RS > SRH); MC pelvis; pelvis and scapula; both scapulae (shoulders)

Impairments: Decreased lower trunk and hip stability and weight shifting; imbalance of knee muscle activity.

45

Description

To enhance stability, the therapist is in a half-kneeling position in front of the patient. AI and RS are applied in a manner similar to that previously described in the quadruped and bridging activities. The uniqueness of this application relates to the position of kneeling. In kneeling the BoS is large posteriorly but minimal anteriorly. Therefore, resistance in the anterior direction must be greatly reduced. To maintain the position the patient needs good trunk control. To assist with stability, the patient's hands can be positioned on the therapist's knee or shoulders. With MCs on the pelvis, AI in the A-P direction is performed (Fig. 45A). Because of the decreased BoS anteriorly, the patient will respond with postural responses in the back and hip ex-

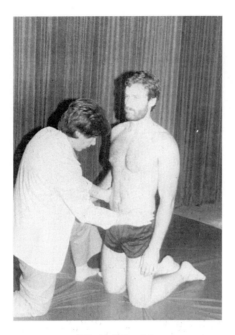

45A AI: MC pelvis.

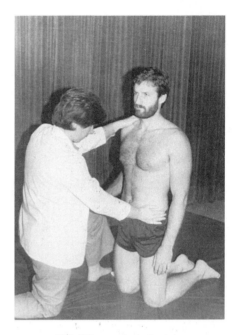

45B MC scapula and pelvis.

tensors, hamstring and ankle muscles when resistance in the anterior direction is applied. AI to M-L is accomplished by positioning MCs on the lateral pelvis. The patient's knees are positioned far enough apart to simulate the position in standing. When AI is applied to rotation, MCs are placed on opposite sides of the pelvis.

For RS the therapist is positioned on the diagonal and can combine approximation with diagonal-rotational resistance. MCs can be placed either on the pelvis, the pelvis and the shoulder (Fig. 45B), both shoulders (Fig. 45C) or the head and the shoulder depending on the area of the body to be emphasized.

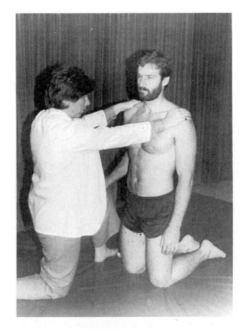

45C MC scapulae.

SRH is usually performed to pelvic motions with MCs placed directly on the pelvis. In the A-P direction, movement occurs through small ranges to promote a balanced interaction of antagonists. This motion occurs both at the knees and the hips with the upper body bending forward as the hips flex. As in bridging, resistance to the flexor motion is difficult, thus full range is not attempted. Similar to bridging, movement in A-P, M-L, and rotational directions will promote the pelvic movements needed for gait. Trunk sidebending toward the weight-bearing side can be combined with weight shifting in the M-L direction.

Purpose/Treatment Goals

The purposes are (1) isometric and isotonic enhancement of pelvic control in the upright position with the lower extremity in an advanced combination of hip extension and knee flexion, (2) enhancement of postural responses during the weight-shifting procedures, and (3) development of proximal dynamic stability in the trunk and hip muscles.

In this procedure the quadriceps may be inhibited by the amount of body weight resistance, the weight bearing on the tendon, and the prolonged stretch. For patients with quadriceps hypertonicity this may be desirable. Because of these inhibitory influences on the quadriceps this kneeling position is included toward the end of the rehabilitation process for patients with quadriceps weakness. If pressure on the knee is uncomfortable, a pillow or foam can be placed under the knees. In kneeling, the sole of the foot is not in contact with the supporting surface, thus kneeling may be easier to maintain for some patients than the hooklying or bridging activities.

To facilitate the movement of kneeling from heel sitting, the trunk flexion pattern of a chop (initial range) and a trunk extension pattern, the lift (completion of the range) may prove helpful. Kneeling also can be assumed from the quadruped position.

Problems with Application

The therapist may have difficulty grading resistance and stretch in the A-P direction.

Because the patient's upper trunk is free to move, total body movements rather than isolated lower trunk motions frequently occur, especially during the lateral and rotational movements. The therapist needs to be aware of this common total body substitution. Positioning the patient's hands on the therapist's shoulders will help stabilize the upper trunk and prevent this movement. If the patient is unable to isolate lower trunk motions even with the upper trunk stabilized, a return to lower level posture, such as sidelying, LTR, and bridging may be indicated.

Activity: Kneeling to heel sitting
Technique: Agonistic reversals (AR); MCs pelvis
Impairments: Decreased eccentric control of hip and knee extensors.

46

Description

Agonistic reversals performed in kneeling will enhance control primarily in the quadriceps and to a lesser extent in the hip extensors. The therapist is in front of the patient with MCs on the anterior pelvis so that resistance can be directed in the posterior direction. The technique is applied through increments of range to gradually increase the quadriceps inhibition that occurs in the lengthened range. The additional inhibitory influences of weight bearing on the quadriceps tendon and the resistance of body weight will add to the difficulty of this procedure. During the eccentric movement into heel sitting the patient's upper body should flex forward to alter the

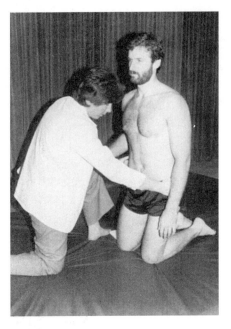

46A AR: Concentric extensors.

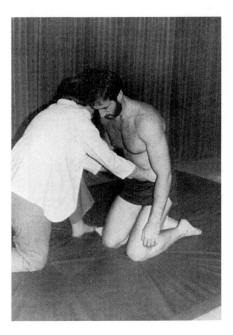

46B AR: Eccentric extensors.

CoG anteriorly and decrease the stress on the quadriceps. With MCs remaining on the anterior surface of the pelvis, verbal commands are "make me work at pushing you down, now come back up to kneeling, now slowly move down toward your heels" (Figs. 46A, 46B).

To increase the activation of the quadriceps the hips may be held in extension throughout the movement, which will shift the CoG posteriorly and greatly increase the stress of the procedure. This more difficult movement may be appropriate for athletes or other patients returning to a very active life.

Purpose/Treatment Goals

The purpose is to increase the eccentric control in the lower extremity extensors, primarily the quadriceps. Because of the numerous inhibitory influences on the quadriceps, this procedure is not usually included until the later stages of rehabilitation of a patient with knee dysfunction. This procedure is appropriate for patients demonstrating difficulty descending stairs due to poor eccentric quadriceps control.

Problems with Application

The challenge may be too great for the patient if full range is attempted initially or if the upper body does not flex anteriorly as heel sitting is achieved.

Activity: Kneeling from quadruped
Technique: Transitional guided movements; MC as needed
Impairments: Difficulty coordinating flexor and extensor movements between the lower trunk and lower extremities; decreased dynamic stability; decreased ability to weight shift through wide ranges.

47

Description

Movement between postures usually follows weight shifting within the posture. Kneeling is frequently assumed from the quadruped position. As with the assumption of most postures there is a flexion and an extension phase. The patient initially bends toward the on-heels position then extends the upper trunk in the second phase to assume the kneeling position. MCs on the upper trunk can assist or guide the patient during these two phases. A rotational motion can be added to both of these phases if the patient seems to be dominated by symmetrical patterns.

Purpose/Treatment Goals

The purpose is to assist the patient in transitional movements from the quadruped to the kneeling postures.

Problems with Application

The patient may overemphasize the flexion phase and actually sit on heels. The CoG is then so posteriorly placed that the patient may have difficulty initiating the extension phase. If, however, the patient does not flex sufficiently, the CoG may be too anterior to allow for a smooth transition between the postures.

Activity: Half-kneeling from kneeling
Technique: Transitional guided movement; MC upper trunk
Impairments: Difficulty controlling trunk balance and rotation with a reduced BoS and moving CoG.

48

Description

The movement to half-kneeling from kneeling incorporates lateral weight shifting, trunk counterrotation, and hip flexion. To facilitate these motions the therapist can stand behind the patient and place MCs on the upper trunk. If the patient displays associated reactions in the limbs, then the placement of MCs can be modified and additional assistance provided to help control tone in these extremities.

The transitional movement begins with lateral weight shifting toward the non-moving lower extremity. The upper body is then rotated and the lower trunk follows with rotation and hip flexion of the moving limb. As the foot contacts the floor, weight is shifted forward onto that foot.

Purpose/Treatment Goals

The purposes are: to assist the patient in moving from kneeling to the half-kneeling position, and to enhance weight shifting and transitional movements.

Problems with Application

The patient may attempt to lift the leg prior to the trunk weight shifting and rotational postural adjustments. If the patient has difficulty with certain phases of this transitional movement, the therapist should include in treatment the specific components of the total pattern that were described during the controlled mobility procedures. For example, lateral weight shifting and rotation can be performed individually before being combined in this transitional motion.

49

Activity: Half-kneeling

Technique: Rhythmic stabilization (RS); slow reversal (SR); MC pelvis

Impairments: Decreased postural stability on the weight-bearing limb; decreased control of knee and ankle flexion.

Description

For most patients, half-kneeling presents the greatest challenge of all the mat activities. The amount of resistance and excursion of movements, therefore, must be carefully graded. Half-kneeling is difficult due to the amount of weight bearing on the posterior limb and the narrowed diagonal BoS. In kneeling the BoS is symmetrical; in half-kneeling support is in a diagonal direction. Resistance and all the patient's movements must occur in the direction of the patient's BoS. The patient's ability to maintain the position is enhanced by the isometric techniques of AI and RS. SR through increments of range can then promote controlled movement (Figs. 49A, 49B). Similar to the A-P movements in kneeling, the patient flexes the upper trunk while moving the pelvis backward.

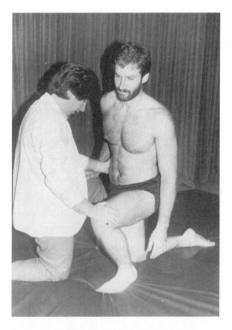

49A Weight shifting forward.

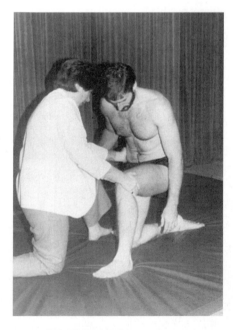

49B Weight shifting backward.

Purpose/Treatment Goals

The purposes are: to promote stability and controlled mobility in half kneeling; to further enhance quadriceps control; to improve both static and dynamic weight-bearing ability of the posterior limb; and to promote movement through range in the knee and foot of the anterior limb.

The three inhibitory influences of body weight resistance, pressure on the quadriceps tendon, and maintained stretch of the muscle challenge the quadriceps control. These inhibitory influences may be maximized in the posterior weight-bearing limb.

This procedure can be incorporated into the treatment plan to facilitate motions of the anterior limb. When rocking forward the ankle is dorsiflexing. This movement can help promote increased talotibial motion because the gastrocnemius is slack at the knee. The knee of the anterior limb is subjected to fewer inhibitory influences as compared with the posterior limb. For patients complaining of pain when weight bearing on the knee, this anterior non-weight-bearing position can be used to develop control at approximately 90 degrees of knee flexion.

Half-kneeling is also useful when teaching a patient how to assume standing or sitting from a lying position. From the half-kneeling position the patient can move into a chair or can lean forward over the anterior limb to assume standing.

Problems with Application

Therapists may incorrectly resist or attempt to move the patient in the diagonal direction in which there is no BoS.

Too much manual resistance is frequently provided during the rocking motions. The resistance of body weight is sufficient to challenge most patients.

Upright Progression

ACTIVITIES

Sitting
Modified plantigrade
Standing

FACTORS RELATING TO THE PROGRESSION OF ACTIVITIES

Biomechanical Factors

Base of support decreases
Center of gravity (mass) elevates
Resistance
  Elongated lever arm lower extremities
  Manual contacts can be altered
  Effects of gravity and weight bearing increased

Reflexive Factors

Tonic influences minimized
Need for postural control maximized

50

Activity: Sitting with or without UE support

Technique: Alternating isometrics progressing to rhythmic stabilization (AI > RS): MC scapula (shoulders; scapula and head)

Impairments: Decreased postural stability of trunk, neck, head and upper body; decreased stability of scapula, glenohumeral, elbow and wrist joints; decreased strength in trunk and upper body muscles.

Mobility	Stability	Controlled Mobility	Skill
Sitting	Alternating isometrics Rhythmic stabilization		

Description

This procedure can be performed to enhance stability of either the trunk or the upper extremities. If trunk control is the goal, the progression begins with the upper extremities supporting. The assistance proved by this increased BoS is gradually reduced. If the procedure is to enhance stability in the upper extremities, then weight bearing through the arms is maintained.

The therapist can be positioned in front of or behind the patient in line with the resistive force. The patient can be long sitting (Fig. 50A) or sitting on a plinth or chair with the feet supported on the floor or stool to assist with stability. The technique of AI can be applied in the A-P, M-L, and rotational directions with moderate and rhythmic resistance to enhance postural stability. MCs are on the appropriate surfaces for application of resistance in the different directions.

RS combines diagonal and rotational resistance to enhance postural stability. MCs are positioned on the superior shoulder region. Diagonal resistance provided by one MC combines A-P and M-L directions with a counterrotational force applied with the other MC. Approximation accompanies these stability techniques unless the patient has disc involvement, osteoporosis, or painful or unstable conditions for which approximation might be contraindicated.

Resistance proved by MCs positioned on the head and the scapula (shoulder) may be used

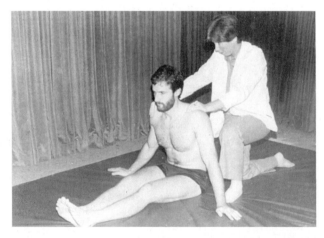

50A Long sitting pictured.

as in P on E, to enhance stability of the head and neck or may be used as an indirect means of activating the musculature of the opposite limb.

Purpose/Treatment Goals

The purposes are to: facilitate postural stability of the musculature around the head and neck, the trunk, the shoulder girdle, and the upper extremities; promote righting reactions of the head and develop static balance responses; and enhance overflow to the LEs primarily to the hip and knee musculature.

Postural control comprises the motor responses of the head, neck, trunk, and extremities to various sensory inputs including visual, vestibular, proprioceptive, and tactile. Static balance, stability, is usually promoted before dynamic balance, controlled mobility. Functional independence or skill in a posture requires dynamic balance and protective extension control.

If in sitting the feet are unsupported, overflow to the legs may be more evident and be seen as normal associated movements. This indirect activation may be the purpose of the procedure.

With the trunk in an upright position, the effects of the tonic reflexes are minimized and gravitational forces are balanced. Sitting, therefore, is an effective position initially to enhance head and neck control prior to the prone progression. Stability of the head and the neck is prerequisite for the vital functions of swallowing and feeding. Frequently patients are positioned in sitting before they have the ability to independently maintain the position. These stability techniques applied to the trunk and the head may assist the patient toward the goal of independent sitting.

Prior to performing these stability techniques, proper sitting alignment needs to be achieved. The pelvis is positioned in midline or in slight anterior tilt which may also improve the lumbar and thoracic alignment. The head is in a midposition avoiding an extreme forward head position. The lower extremities are positioned in neutral in relation to rotation and abduction–adduction. For patients with pain associated with spinal compression, weight bearing through the trunk may increase symptoms. If this occurs, altering alignment or diffusing weight bearing by pelvic tilting, altering the lumbar curve, or sitting on a foam pad or ball may alleviate pain in the early stages. For those with excessive kyphosis, stability in an erect position is indicated to improve the endurance of the upper back extensors. Hold relax to the anterior chest muscles combined with breathing patterns emphasizing inspiration may be used prior to these stability techniques to improve alignment.

In sitting, the shoulder is in the least painful position of approximately zero degrees of flexion. Small amounts of weight bearing through the arm is effective in facilitating scapular stability and the rotator cuff musculature in the early stages of treatment for patients with shoulder dysfunction. The weight-bearing upper extremities can be placed anterior, posterior, or lateral to the hips of the patient depending on indications for weight bearing and positioning.

Weight bearing occurs through the elbow in the shortened range of extension, which is an important position for hemiplegic patients. The hand is in contact with the supporting surface that can have an inhibitory influence on the finger flexors.

In sitting, stability of the upper trunk can be performed. With the upper extremities non-weight bearing and positioned in D1E or in a D1 withdrawal pattern, thoracic extension can be combined with scapular adduction and depression, and shoulder extension. A shortened held resisted contraction can be resisted manually, with pulleys or an elastic band. This procedure is indicated for patients with excessive kyphosis, weakness, fatigue or "burning" in the thoracic musculature, or poor stability in the scapular musculature.

Long sitting is an important posture in the rehabilitation of patients with spinal cord injury, and developing stability in the long sitting posture is a prerequisite to other functional activities.

Problems with Application

The therapist may easily overpower the patient. As in all postures, resistance needs to be applied gradually to appropriately match and not overcome holding by the patient.

51

Activity: Sitting; upper trunk motions

Technique: Slow reversal hold through increments of range (SRH): MC scapula

Impairments: Decreased dynamic balance; decreased ability to reverse antagonists; dominance of abnormal flexor or extensor tone; decreased weight bearing on one side of the body; decreased or asymmetric sensory feedback from the trunk.

Mobility	Stability	Controlled Mobility	Skill
Sitting		Slow reversal hold	
Trunk movements			

Description

The controlled mobility level of motor control for the trunk in sitting is weight shifting or upper trunk flexion and extension with rotation. The therapist is diagonally anterior to the patient and MCs are positioned on the anterior upper trunk to facilitate trunk flexion with rotation. The commands are "look down, bend your trunk and bring your right shoulder down toward your left knee." The combined motion of trunk flexion with rotation is resisted with both MCs. In the shortened range of the movement an isometric contraction is performed (Fig. 51A), followed by a gentle stretch to the antagonistic extensors. The verbal commands are "look up and over your opposite shoulder and sit up straight" as resistance is applied to extension with rotation (Fig. 51B). The verbal commands are important to ensure that the head movement leads the trunk motions.

Active movements can be performed to teach the patient how to control changes in the center of mass.

Purpose/Treatment Goals

The purposes are to: (1) promote controlled mobility and weight shifting in the sitting position, (2) facilitate righting and dynamic balance responses, and (3) enhance the patient's ability to assume sitting as movements through increments of range are achieved.

If the patient has difficulty with postural control responses the therapist must differentially assess the sensory and motor systems. Sensations that contribute to balance are visual, vestibular, proprioceptive, and tactile. Diminished input can alter the awareness of motion and can lead to diminished motor responses. Both static and dynamic motor responses need to be evaluated.

In sitting, the small BoS and high CoG may challenge postural responses to the extent that movement through a large range is difficult. Trunk flexion is assisted by gravity; therefore this activity is appropriate for patients with poor abdominal strength. For patients with parkinsonism the rotational motion can be isolated by positioning the MCs on opposite sides of the trunk.

With the patient's hands and feet in contact with a supporting surface, such as a ball, small amounts of movement in the extremities as well as alterations in weight bearing can be pro-

bility may be associated with diminished proprioceptive awareness and decreased ability to maintain postural stability. These prior stages of control need to be remediated by appropriate procedures (Procedures 17, 41, and 120).

Activity: Sitting; diagonal movements of one UE

Technique: Slow reversal (SR), guided or active movement; MC supporting scapula and dynamic arm

Impairments: Decreased postural control in the trunk; decreased proximal dynamic stability; decreased control over trunk rotation; decreased ability to control weight shifting in the trunk and hips.

53

	Mobility	Stability	Controlled Mobility	Static Dynamic	Skill
Sitting				Slow reversal,	
Limb				guided or active	
movement				movement	

Description

Movements of the dynamic limb can be performed in the D1 or D2 patterns or in any direction which appropriately challenges trunk control (Fig. 53A). The amount of resistance provided to the dynamic limb and the amount of range through which the arm moves is dependent on the control of the static parts. The therapist can be positioned either in front of or behind the patient, whichever affords the best control. The MC on the dynamic limb is on the forearm, not

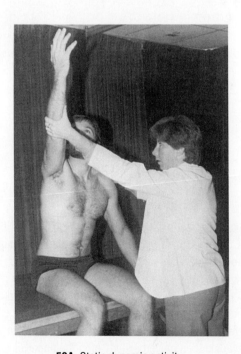

53A Static dynamic activity.

more distally, as specific control of the dynamic limb is not usually the goal of the procedure. The patient can perform the procedure independently using an elastic band, a cuff weight, or any weighted object.

Purpose/Treatment Goals

The purposes are to further develop postural responses in the trunk; enhance weight shifting; and promote movement in the trunk, dynamic limb, and weight-bearing scapula and shoulder.

Static–dynamic activities can be performed to further challenge trunk control by reducing the BoS or may be used to promote proximal control of the static, weight-bearing scapula.

This procedure is appropriate for hemiplegic patients or patients with painful shoulder dysfunction. Dynamic-stability control is promoted in the weight-bearing limb in a position of minimal challenge. Patients with weakness of scapular muscles may find this procedure useful. The movement between the weight-bearing scapula and the thorax is produced by active motion of the trunk beneath the relatively fixed scapula. This active mobilization is an indirect method to initiate movement in a painful part.

The trunk movements that accompany the limb patterns can be useful for patients with scoliosis or other trunk abnormalities.

Problems with Application

The therapist may apply too much resistance to the dynamic arm. Observation of the responses in the trunk and static limb will provide the therapist with feedback regarding the appropriate amount of resistance to be applied to the dynamic arm.

54

Activity: Sitting; dynamic balance

Technique: Active guided movement; MC scapula or distal UE

Impairments: Decreased dynamic balance; diminished sensory input; decreased ability to quickly reverse antagonists.

Mobility	Stability	Controlled Mobility	Skill
Sitting			Active guided movement

Description

Righting reactions and postural control responses can be facilitated by gentle and slow disturbances of the patient's CoG or BoS while the patient is seated on a raised mat or in a chair. The feet can be supported to provide additional assistance or left free to increase the challenge to trunk control. The patient can self displace the CoG several ways: by reaching with an upper extremity in all directions, for example bending forward to reach toward the feet, or lifting one leg. The challenge can be increased by increasing the excursion, lifting contralateral limbs and sitting on an unstable surface, for example, a ball. The therapist can challenge control with MCs first positioned on the scapula then moved distally onto the upper or lower limbs to increase the length of the lever arm and increase the number of segments involved. Postural control can be disturbed in A-P, M-L, diagonal and rotational directions. Trunk rotation can be combined with lateral shifting and occur at the initiation of or after the shift. These variations may alter abdominal or trunk extensor activity and the responses of the lower extremities. The desired responses are righting of the head and appropriate postural responses in the trunk and the extremities depending on the direction of displacement. As control is gained, the excursion and speed of motion may be increased.

Purpose/Treatment Goals

The purposes are to facilitate righting and dynamic postural responses in the sitting position, and encourage functional movement of the upper extremities in the posture.

Problems with Application

Therapists may attempt this procedure too early in the rehabilitation process. To successfully respond to disturbances of the CoG or BoS, postural control and sufficient strength need to be present as well as the sensory awareness of the changing CoG. If the patient has difficulty responding, the therapist must evaluate both the sensory and motor systems to determine the area of deficit.

Summary

If the goal is to develop trunk control, the progression begins with a large BoS, both UEs and LEs supporting. The BoS is then reduced as static–dynamic activities are performed. Self-displacement activities, i.e., reaching for an object, simulates the functional control the patient needs in sitting. This can then be followed by balancing on an unstable surface such as a balance board or ball.

Activity: Sitting; upper trunk motions with the cradling position
Technique: Slow reversal hold (SRH), slow reversal (SR), or guided movement; MC on elbows
Impairments: Decreased postural control in the trunk; stiffness and decreased ability to initiate movement in the proximal upper extremities.

55

Description

In sitting, upper trunk or proximal upper extremity motions can be facilitated by crossing the upper extremities in the cradling position. The movement of the trunk and limbs is guided by the therapist who is sitting and facing the patient. MCs are positioned on the elbows. The motions can be performed in individual planes of trunk flexion-extension and rotation or these trunk motions can be combined. Depending on the treatment goals the focus can be on the trunk motion or on the proximal scapular and shoulder movements.

Purpose/Treatment Goals

The purposes are to facilitate weight shifting in sitting and to promote proximal motion of the scapula and the shoulder. The length of the lever arm is relatively short and there are few joints involved in this activity when compared with other trunk patterns (reverse chop and prayer position). This procedure, therefore, may be appropriate when initially facilitating upper extremity mobility.

Problems with Application

The cradling position is similar to the abnormal resting position of the hemiplegic limb. For patients with hemiplegia, this cradling position may be appropriate only during early stages when pain or primitive patterns limit other voluntary control.

56

Activity: Sitting; upper trunk extension pattern (lift)
Technique: Slow reversal hold (SRH); rhythmic stabilization (RS)
Impairments: Diminished dynamic balance; decreased proximal upper extremity control; decreased trunk rotation or extension.

Description

Because the patient's two upper extremities are non-weight bearing and moving with the distal segment free, this activity performed with SRH is considered at the skill level of movement control. The lifting pattern promotes trunk extension with rotation. The procedure is most easily controlled with the patient sitting in a chair or on a raised mat with feet supported.

The therapist may be positioned behind the patient in the diagonal direction of the pattern. With one MC on the head and the other on the wrist of the lead D2F arm, the patient is passively moved through the lifting pattern before resistance is applied.

To perform the technique of SRH, a stretch is applied in the lengthened range of the pattern (Fig. 56A), followed by resistance through range with an isometric hold applied in the shortened range (Fig. 56B). The stretch can be enhanced with a traction force and the hold in the shortened range can be facilitated with approximation. The antagonistic pattern is then stretched and only slightly resisted. The emphasis of the procedure is on the lift and not on the reverse lift.

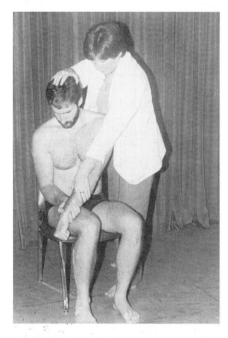

56A Lift: Stretch in lengthened range.

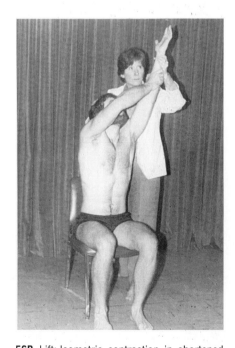

56B Lift: Isometric contraction in shortened range.

To facilitate proximal upper limb or upper trunk stability, RS can be applied at various points in the range. To perform this technique, resistance is applied to the lifting pattern until the range to be emphasized with RS is reached. At this range isometric resistance is applied simultaneously in opposite directions or to antagonistic muscle groups by alternating the direction of resistance on the head and wrist. This isometric resistance is alternated until a moderate level of intensity is achieved. At this point both MCs isometrically resist again in the direction of the lifting movement before an isotonic contraction through more range is allowed. RS can be applied at sequential points throughout the range as indicated.

The patient can perform the movement with resistance provided by pulleys, theraband or any weighted object.

Purpose/Treatment Goals

The purposes are to: (1) facilitate the proximal dynamic stability needed for the skill level of movement control, (2) improve head and trunk extension with rotation in combination with the asymmetrical upper trunk pattern, (3) improve respiration (inspiration with the lift and expiration with the reverse lift), and (4) further challenge trunk control by reducing the BoS. The technique of RS is used with the lift to facilitate upper extremity range and stability.

Patients with burns in the axilla may have limitations in the shoulder motions that occur in D2F. The assistance provided by the other limb in the lift coupled with the technique of RS, that promotes isometric contractions, may increase the amount of range if pain limits movement. The isometric contractions may cause the muscles to move under the skin. If adhesions between these two surfaces have developed, the slight sliding that occurs during the muscle contraction may be beneficial.

The trunk motions of extension and rotation are particularly appropriate for patients with parkinsonism. The lifting motion can be performed independently as part of a home program.

For patients with weakness in the rotator cuff or poor scapular stability, RS performed through increments of range may enhance the muscular control needed during this difficult motion.

Problems with Application

The therapist may be positioned incorrectly and therefore movement into the proper diagonal direction will be difficult. Resistance should be provided to both the head and the upper extremities during RS. Care must be taken, however, so that each part is challenged but not overstressed. The sequencing of the resistive forces with RS may be difficult; the therapist should practice the order beginning with resistance in the agonistic direction, then in alternating directions, then ending in the agonistic direction before movement into the pattern is completed.

57

Activity: Sitting; trunk flexion pattern (chop)

Technique: Timing for emphasis (TE); slow reversal hold (SRH); MC head and wrist

Impairments: Decreased ability to shift weight laterally and forward; decreased strength of upper abdominal muscles; decreased trunk flexion with rotation.

Desciption

This procedure, that can also be considered to promote the skill stage of control, promotes trunk flexion with rotation. This upper trunk motion was first promoted during the controlled mobility procedure in sitting with the patient's upper extremities weight bearing and the therapist's MCs on the trunk. The upper trunk activity of a chop is more difficult because the limbs are not in contact with the surface and therefore do not assist with balance. In addition, the therapist's MCs are more distal, involving more joints and creating a longer lever arm. An advantage of this upper trunk procedure is the promotion of overflow from stronger head and UE muscles into weaker upper abdominal musculature and to the lower extremities.

The patient is positioned short sitting in a chair or on a plinth; the feet may be supported. The therapist is positioned diagonally in front of the plinth and close to the side of the patient. Once MC is on the head and one on the wrist of the lead D1 limb. During SRH, resistance is provided to both the flexion and extension directions, i.e., the chop (Fig. 57A) and reverse chop (Fig. 57B). However, emphasis is placed on the trunk flexion motion. Verbal commands are "tuck your chin and open your hand and bring your arms down toward your knee, hold it, now look up and over your shoulder and bring your arms up toward the ceiling."

If the goal is to strengthen the abdominals, TE can be performed in the shortened range of the chop. To perform TE, the stronger head and extremity segments are resisted to their shortened range where they are "locked in" with isometric resistance and an approximation force. Once the hold can be maintained in the stronger segments (head and extremities), the focus is

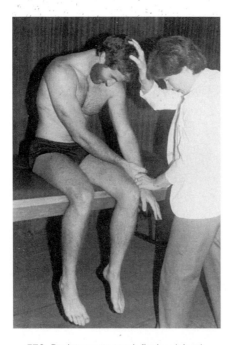

57A Resistance to trunk flexion (chop).

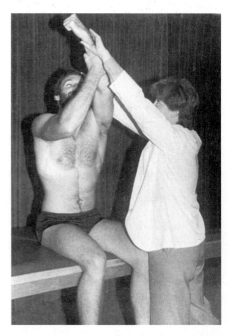

57B Resistance to trunk extension (reverse chop).

changed to the trunk where the abdominal contraction is facilitated by stretch and resistance. The direction of the stretch and resistive force is toward the opposite shoulder in the direction of the upper abdominals.

Purpose/Treatment Goals

The purposes are to facilitate weight shifting and strengthen the upper abdominal muscles.

Because trunk flexion is assisted by gravity, the trunk flexion motion in sitting is appropriate for muscles below a 3/5 grade. Resistance, however, must be sufficient to counteract the effects of gravity. A progression from this sitting position would be to supine where the abdominals would be flexing the trunk against gravity.

This procedure may be appropriate for patients with paraparesis. If sitting balance is lacking, the trunk flexion pattern may have to be performed in sidelying or supine and resistance adjusted to counter the effects of gravity.

The procedure may be used for patients with hemiparesis. Goals may include crossing of the midline, movement of the UE out of synergistic patterns, and weight shifting over the involved side. Resistance must be carefully graded to avoid enhancing abnormal movements.

In this procedure overflow to the lower extremities may be noted and this may be the goal of the procedure. Resistance also can be applied by pulleys or an elastic band.

Problems with Application

Therapists may have difficulty applying resistance in the diagonal direction. If too much resistance is given in the initial and midrange of the chop, the patient may tend to move the extremities in a circular "windmill" movement. The therapist must guide the extremities in the correct pattern of movement in line with the oblique fibers of the abdominals.

During the TE technique the head and limbs must be resisted into their shortened range before being "locked in." The trunk flexion movement is then emphasized. Frequently a therapist allows excessive trunk flexion before beginning TE and thus facilitates hip flexion.

With the patient sitting on a plinth, the therapist may have difficulty controlling the shortened range of the reverse chop. Because this is not the direction usually emphasized during this procedure, movement into this range may intentionally be limited.

....

Activity: Sitting; D1 thrust assisted, BS D1 thrust and withdrawal patterns

Technique: Shortened held resisted contraction (SHRC); slow reversal hold (SRH); guided movement; MC wrists

Impairments: Decreased scapular stability; weakness serratus anterior, middle trapezius, rhomboids, anterior and posterior deltoid, rotator cuff, biceps and triceps; weakness and poor endurance in thoracic extensors; decreased initiation of glenohumeral movement.

58

Description

The therapist is positioned in front of the patient with MCs on the wrists. The withdrawal pattern performed bilaterally in sitting can be used as a modified pivot prone–prone extension activity (Fig. 58A). A SHRC in the shortened range of the withdrawal pattern is used to facilitate trunk and scapular muscle stability. The primary muscles facilitated are the upper trunk exten-

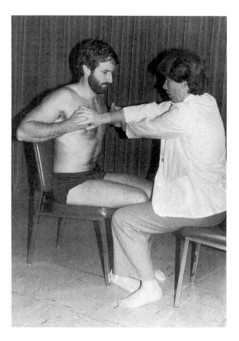

58A BSD1 withdrawal.

sors, middle trapezius, rhomboids, and the posterior deltoids. With the technique of SRH, both directions of the pattern can be resisted.

Purpose/Treatment Goals

The purpose is to facilitate muscle stability in the upper trunk and proximal upper extremities. This position is appropriate for patients who cannot assume the pivot prone posture. When performed as reversing motions, the procedure facilitates proximal control, trunk balance, and is a

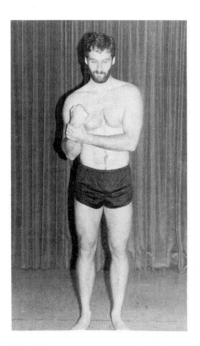

58B D1 thrust-assisted lengthened range.

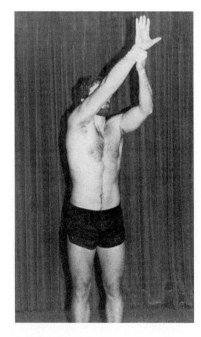

58C Shortened range.

progression from movements performed in supine. In sitting, the support which was provided to the scapula in supine is absent increasing the difficulty of the movement. The thrust also may be performed as a trunk pattern (Figs. 58B, 58C) and can be used to facilitate hand opening above 90 degrees. Both movements can easily be performed as part of a home program for patients with shoulder dysfunction.

Problems with Application

In the shortened range of the thrusting pattern, the shoulder should be flexed above 90 degrees. The therapist may inappropriately limit this range and thus overemphasize horizontal adduction and abduction.

Activity: Sitting; upper extremity, bilateral symmetrical D2F (UE BS D2F)

Technique: Slow reversal hold; MC arms

Impairments: Decreased thoracic or lumbar extension or excessive thoracic kyphosis; diminished inspiratory volume; weakness in the lower trapezius, middle deltoid and rotator cuff muscles; decreased trunk postural control.

59

Description

Because the upper extremities are not in contact with each other this procedure is often more difficult than the trunk patterns of lift and chop. The shoulder flexion pattern is accompanied by trunk extension and inspiration; shoulder extension is combined with trunk flexion and expiration. The therapist can be positioned either in front of or behind the patient. In an anterior position the therapist can best control the lengthened ranges of D2F or the shortened range of D2E; posteriorly the shortened ranges of D2F or the lengthened range of D2E can be best controlled (Fig. 59A). MCs

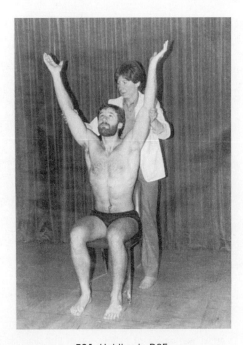

59A Holding in D2F.

may need to be on the proximal forearms or on the upper arm so that greater ranges of scapular and shoulder movement can be resisted. Resistance also can be provided by pulleys, an elastic band or any weighted object.

Purpose/Treatment Goals

The purposes are to facilitate the skill level of control in the trunk and the proximal upper extremity musculature; facilitate trunk extension or flexion motions; and promote breathing patterns. Patients with excessive kyphosis may improve upper trunk extension by performing this procedure.

Problems with Application

MCs may be incorrectly positioned distally, preventing full range of proximal movement. Patients with restricted scapular motion or decreased rotator cuff control may experience pain in the lateral shoulder. Movement and control may need to be promoted into D1F prior to D2F.

60

Activity: Sitting; D2 thrust (flexor and extensor synergy–rowing); bilateral and unilateral

Technique: Slow reversal hold (SRH); timing emphasis (TE); MC wrists

Impairments: Inability to initiate any movement of the upper extremity; prolonged flaccidity following a CVA.

Description

In sitting, the synergistic patterns of the upper extremity can be facilitated by enhancing overflow from the less involved limb. The proximal component of shoulder movements is similar in

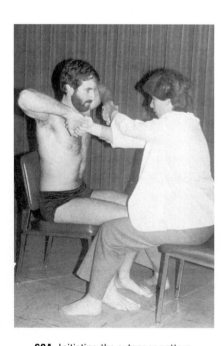

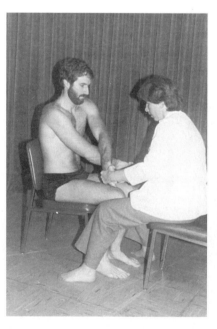

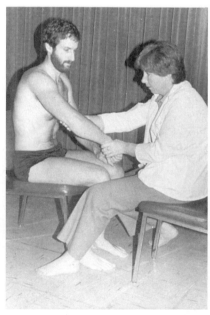

60A Initiating the extensor pattern.

60B Holding in shortened range of extensor pattern.

60C Facilitating triceps response.

both the D2 thrust and the synergistic pattern. If the movement is performed as a bilateral combination, TE can be used to enhance overflow from one limb to the other. If facilitation of a specific component of the pattern, e.g., elbow extension, is a goal, a unilateral pattern may be a better choice. During the performance of unilateral patterns both of the therapist's contacts are on the involved limb and thus can be used to better emphasize a particular segment.

The therapist sits in front of the patient. If the pattern is performed bilaterally to initiate proximal activity, MCs are on both wrists (Figs. 60A, 60B). If a unilateral pattern is chosen to enhance elbow motion then MCs are on the upper arm and the wrist (Fig. 60C).

Purpose/Treatment Goals

The purpose is to facilitate synergistic patterns in the upper extremity for hemiplegic patients who remain at a flaccid stage for a prolonged time. Those who have a dominant flexor synergy may benefit from the facilitation of the extensor pattern.

Problems with Applications

The rowing pattern will enhance the synergistic patterns. If the patient can independently initiate synergistic movements the goal would be to recombine movement combinations by enhancing D1F and D2F as previously described. Therapists may incorrectly guide the shoulder into extension during the flexor phase rather than facilitating shoulder flexion and abduction with external rotation.

Activity: Sitting; unilateral LE flexion
Technique: Assisted movement; hold after positioning; hold relax active movement; MC thigh and foot
Impairments: Inability to initiate any flexion motion in the lower extremity; dominance of extensor tone in the leg.

61

Description

In sitting, the lower extremity is in a mass flexion position. To facilitate flexion of the lower extremity the therapist may guide the leg into more flexion, then promote holding in shortened ranges with the technique of hold after positioning. Once hip flexion is achieved (Fig. 61A), then knee flexion (Fig. 61B) is promoted with the therapist guiding the patient's foot under the chair. Flexion of the ankle can be facilitated in this mass flexion position before the procedure is made more difficult by extending the hip and the knee (Fig. 61C). With hold relax active movement, movement is facilitated from a slightly stretched position after the shortened range has been emphasized.

Purpose/Treatment Goals

The purpose is to initiate hip, knee, and ankle flexion in patients who may have a dominance of extensor tone. Performing these flexor movements may be easier in this sitting posture with a progression to supine.

Problems with Application

Patients with stiffness in the posterior hip structures may have difficulty with the range required.

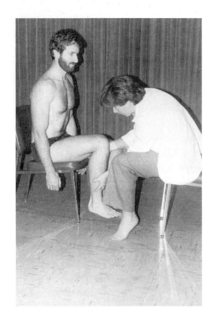

61A Hip flexion.

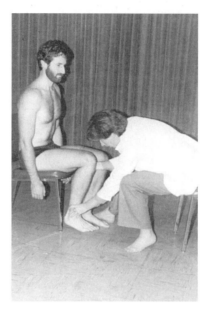

61B Knee flexion.

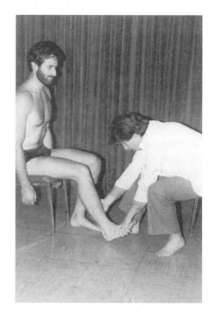

61C Dorsiflexion.

62

Activity: Modified plantigrade; LE symmetrical position and in stride

Technique: Alternating isometrics (AI); rhythmic stabilization (RS); slow reversal hold (SRH) (AI > RS > SRH); static–dynamic activities; MC pelvis; pelvis and scapula; scapula and arm; knee

Impairments: Decreased stability and dynamic stability in the trunk, hips, knees, ankles, shoulders, and elbows; imbalance of flexor and extensor musculature; tendency toward hyperextension of knees or elbows; poor eccentric control gastrocnemius-soleus; osteoporosis, or osteopenia in trunk or upper extremities.

Description

All four limbs are weight bearing, therefore stability and controlled mobility can be promoted in all weight-bearing joints in this easily assumed position. The focus of this discussion is on the clinical application of these procedures, as the techniques have been previously practiced in many other postures.

The lower extremity is in the advanced combination of hip flexion with the knee extended. Advanced combinations are appropriate for hemiplegic patients when the goal of the procedure is to recombine synergistic movements. Knee flexion in this position can be facilitated first with the hip in more flexion, that can be gradually reduced as control is gained.

Weight bearing occurs through the ankle. For patients with reduced postural control, especially during the stance phase of gait, this progression of techniques can promote both stability and controlled mobility at the foot and the ankle. Resistance can be applied and movement can occur in all directions. Weight shifting with the feet in a stride position will simulate the distal control needed during the stance phase of ambulation. For those patients with hypertonia in the gastrocnemius-soleus, weight shifting can facilitate the eccentric control needed in these posterior muscles and thus help reduce the tendency to hyperextend the knee in stance. The stress on the ankle musculature can be progressed from a bilateral weight-bearing position to unilat-

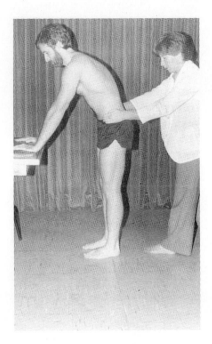

62A AI, RS with MC pelvis.

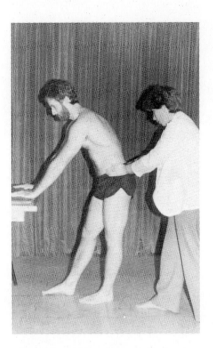

62B SRH weight-shifting posterior leg; promoting ROM proximal UE.

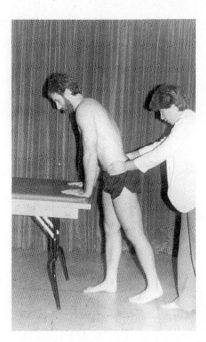

62C SRH weight-shifting anterior leg; promoting weight-bearing UE.

eral weight bearing on the involved limb, to weight bearing on a balance board bilaterally then unilaterally. Weight bearing can be concentrated either on the heel (ankle dorsiflexed) or on the forefoot (ankle plantarflexed). Within this progression, stability is challenged with isometric resistance (Fig. 62A) and controlled mobility with weight shifting in different directions (Figs. 62B, 62C).

The knee is maintained in the shortened range of extension, which is appropriate for patients with weak quadriceps. As a progression, more weight can be accepted onto the involved limb and slight knee flexion can be added. MCs can be placed above and below the knee to more directly promote hamstring and quadriceps stability and controlled movement. For patients with weakness of the hamstrings maintaining the knee extended, but not hyperextended is important. AI with MC at the knee can enhance stability in this range and also increase awareness of the position. Short arc quadriceps and hamstring exercises can be resisted by pulleys or an elastic band (Procedure 147).

The low back is not in the extreme of either flexion or extension. Many patients with low back dysfunction will assume this position when performing activities of daily living such as brushing teeth or shaving. Postural stability in the lower trunk area can be facilitated with the technique of RS. Gentle movements in all directions are promoted with SRH. Patients with low back pain associated with spinal stenosis may experience symptomatic relief in this position. Treatment can encourage segmental opening to further relieve pain. Lifting one limb then contralateral limbs will promote trunk stability and is less difficult than the similar exercise performed in quadruped.

Scapular and shoulder dynamic stability can be facilitated with the shoulder in about 45 to 60 degrees of flexion. Isometric stability with RS is followed by rocking in diagonal directions to promote movement and dynamic stability in the D1 or D2 patterns. MCs can be placed on the upper body to directly challenge UE control. Patients with shoulder dysfunction should move so that the involved limb moves first in the D1 pattern, then progress to D2. This progression pro-

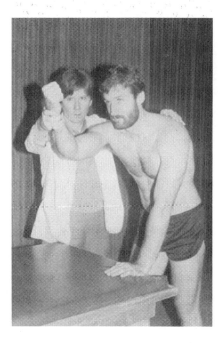

62D Static–dynamic activities increasing weight-bearing and postural responses.

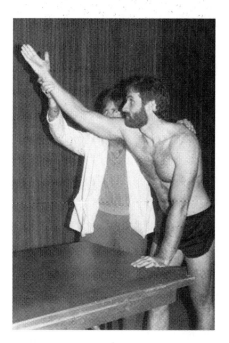

62E Movement into D2F and thoracic extension

motes a gradual increase in the amount of weight bearing through the limb and range through which the limb moves. Static–dynamic activities will increase weight bearing on the supporting involved limb (Figs. 62D, 62E). The increased body weight-bearing resistance will further challenge the proximal muscles.

At the elbow the triceps is isometrically contracting in the shortened range, an important consideration for patients with weakness or hemiparesis. The wrist and finger flexors are in maintained contact with the surface that is considered an inhibitory influence to these muscles. This inhibition is important for patients with finger flexor spasticity. If the amount of wrist and finger extension range is too stressful for the patient, the hand can be placed over the edge of the plinth; to promote wrist stability weight bearing through a fisted hand can be substituted.

Weight bearing through the wrist promotes contraction of the wrist flexors and extensors. This is appropriate for patients recovering from a wrist fracture or from "tennis elbow." Weight bearing also can be on the fingers, which will improve the control of the intrinsics of the hand.

Modified plantigrade techniques to promote stability, AI and RS, are followed by those to promote controlled mobility, SRH and AR. To increase weight bearing and proximal dynamic stability, static–dynamic procedures are performed. The lower extremities can be positioned in a symmetrical pattern, or in stride.

If weight bearing through the elbow or on the hand or wrist is problematic, the position can be altered to weight bearing on elbows. However, in the on-elbows position the triceps are on stretch and there is weight bearing on the tendon which results in inhibitory influences to the triceps.

An important point to remember is that weight bearing on a joint requires mobility to attain the position, but weight bearing through a joint requires muscular control to maintain the joint position.

Purpose/Treatment Goals

The purposes are to promote stability and dynamic stability in all weight-bearing segments, and to enhance endurance in trunk musculature as static–dynamic positions are maintained.

Problems with Application

Knee hyperextension may occur if patients have weakness in the quadriceps or hamstrings, tightness in the ankle joint or gastrocnemius-soleus, or diminished position sense.

The scapula may excessively lift off the thorax or abduct if there is weakness of the serratus anterior, trapezius, or rhomboids.

Activity: Standing from sitting

Technique: Assist to position; MC as needed

Impairments: Inability to independently assume standing from sitting; decreased strength of back, hip, and knee extensors.

63

	Mobility	Stability	Controlled Mobility	Skill
Standing	Assist to position			

Description

The purpose of this procedure is to assist the patient into the standing position and is usually performed with the patient in a wheelchair or straight-backed chair in the parallel bars or next to some supporting surface such as a plinth or a bed. To assist the patient toward the edge of the seat the therapist stands in front of the patient and places one MC around the patient's back and moves the patient laterally to produce weight shifting onto one hip. The other MC is placed under the thigh of the unweighted limb to assist this limb forward. The therapist then changes MCs to weight shift the trunk in the other direction and assist the other leg forward. Verbal cues are "push your knee forward or twist your hip forward" to promote active pelvic forward rotation. After a few repetitions the patient should be sitting near the edge of the chair.

The patient's lower extremity, which will assume most of the weight, is positioned slightly posterior to the other limb. The weight-bearing knee is blocked by the therapist and one MC is placed on that side posteriorly on the pelvis. The lower trunk is anteriorly tilted and the rest of the trunk follows in the forward direction. The other MC is on the opposite shoulder. A rhythmic trunk flexion and extension movement is begun to initiate momentum. On the count of three the patient is assisted to standing. The patient is stabilized by the therapist's knee blocking the patient's knee and the MC on the pelvis guiding the pelvis forward. The therapist's MC on the upper trunk guides the patient's weight over the weight-bearing limb.

If the patient has a stronger side, weight bearing toward that side is initially performed. Weight bearing onto the more involved side should be encouraged once the stability of the less involved limb is ascertained. To ensure the therapist's safety, the therapist positions one leg posteriorly to increase the BoS.

Purpose/Treatment Goal

The purpose is to assist the patient who cannot independently assume the position. Many patients may be able to maintain standing but not be able to achieve the position without assistance.

Problems with Application

Therapists may attempt to stand the patient without first moving the patient to the edge of the seat. If the patient's CoG is too posterior assumption of standing will be very difficult. In addition, the patient's weight-bearing limb must be positioned slightly posteriorly so that the BoS will be closer to the CoG enabling the patient to stand more easily. Therapists often use both legs to block the patient's knee. Such positioning narrows the therapist's BoS and makes it difficult for the therapist to prevent the patient from falling forward.

64

Activity: Standing; pelvic movements
Technique: Alternating isometrics; rhythmic stabilization; slow reversal hold (AI, RS, SRH); MC pelvis or as needed
Impairments: Decreased stability or dynamic stability in trunk, pelvis, hip, knee, and ankle.

Description

The patient stands with feet slightly apart and symmetrical. With MCs on the pelvis, AI is performed in three directions. RS combines resistance in the three directions to promote simultaneous contraction around the weight-bearing segments (Fig. 64A). In conjunction with these stability techniques, approximation forces are added. MCs also can be placed on other body parts, scapula, and pelvis (Fig. 64B), scapulae, the head and the scapula, or knees as previously described. SRH is performed in the straight planes of movement (A-P, M-L, and rotation) (Fig. 64C). To simulate the pelvic control needed during gait, the feet are positioned in stride and the pelvic motions in all three planes are combined. With MC on the anterior surface of the pelvis, the pelvis of the posterior leg is guided forward, shifted laterally over the anterior weight-bearing limb and rotated forward. During forward rotation of the swing pelvis, the pelvis of the stance side (forward limb) must not be allowed to rotate backward. As the swing pelvis rotates forward the entire trunk may have a tendency to rotate in one direction rather than to counterrotate. If this "log rolling" occurs, more emphasis must be placed first on individual pelvic movements to promote isolated forward pelvic rotation.

Purpose/Treatment Goals

The purposes are to promote the pelvic motions needed during gait and to enhance weight shifting and the dynamic stability of the proximal muscles in preparation for ambulation.

During these procedures control of the stance and swing phase can be promoted. These two phases of gait can be related to the stages of control in the following way: moving forward onto the stance leg and controlling the body weight over the fixed distal foot is similar to controlled mobility; during swing, the distal segment is moving which is representative of skill. For this reason emphasis is placed first on gaining control in the stance phase of gait prior to enhancing the swing phase.

These procedures are appropriate for a multitude of patients including amputees, hemiplegics, or those with hip, knee, or ankle dysfunction. If extremely poor knee or ankle control of

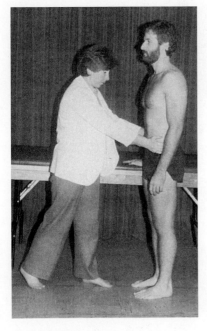
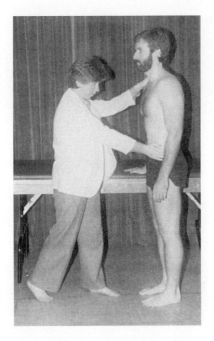
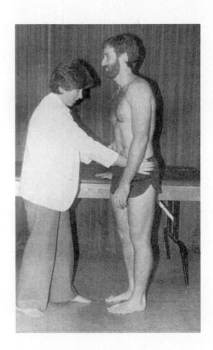

64A AI, RS with MC on pelvis.   **64B** AI, RS with MC scapula and pelvis.   **64C** SRH to pelvic rotation.

one limb interferes with maintaining the position, the patient can kneel with the involved limb on a chair or mat so that pelvic control can be developed.

Problems with Application

The patient may tend to bear weight on a hyperflexed or hyperextended knee. The therapist must be sure that the pelvic and knee positions are consistent with those that occur during gait.

Activity: Standing in stride; forward progression to deliberate walking
Techniques: Resisted progression (RP); MC pelvis
Impairments: Improper timing and sequencing of pelvic movement; decreased ability to weight shift or weight bear during stance.

65

	Mobility	Stability	Controlled Mobility	Skill
Standing		Alternating isometrics Rhythmic stabilization	Slow reversal hold	Resisted progression

Description

The first portion of this procedure as described emphasized the pelvic movement during stance followed by the early swing phases of gait. The involved limb practices weight acceptance and proximal control throughout the stance phase. The timing and sequencing of motion during the swing phase is subsequently promoted.

To continue, the patient's limbs are positioned in stride as in the previous procedure with the more involved leg anterior. With MCs on the pelvis, the movement of the pelvis in a forward

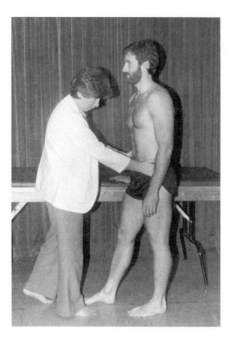

65A Initiating pelvic motions.

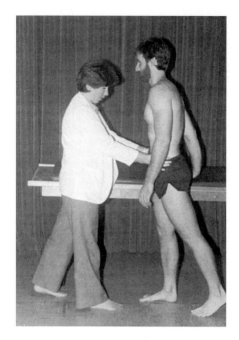

65B Emphasizing pelvic anterior, rotation and lateral shifting motions.

and lateral direction over the stance leg is encouraged (Figs. 65A, 65B). This is combined with forward rotation of the swing pelvis. The pelvis on the stance side remains forward as the swing side is rotated forward. This pelvic motion is emphasized as patients frequently lose control of the stance side as the swing limb begins to rotate. Approximation is applied as weight is accepted onto the stance limb. This portion of the forward progression is repeated until the sequence of pelvic motions is correct.

To focus on the swing phase the involved limb is moved to the posterior position. The swing pelvis is rotated forward while the foot is still in contact with the floor. The swing leg then flexes forward to the heel strike position. Weight is accepted on that leg and an approximation force is simultaneously applied to facilitate limb extension.

Deliberate walking is next and can be performed in the parallel bars or as free walking with the therapist providing support as needed. MCs can be placed on the pelvis. Tracking, guided resistance is applied to facilitate the proper timing and sequencing of the movement. The procedure begins with the feet in stride. Weight is shifted over the forward leg. The pelvis of the swing leg rotates forward as the leg swings through. Weight is shifted forward and over (anterior and lateral) the new stance leg. The progression is continued. The commands may be "shift your weight forward over the left leg, now rotate your right hip forward (stretch to rotation) and bring your right leg through." "Put weight on that leg (approximation through the pelvis) and shift forward and over that leg." A slight stretch, approximation at heel strike, and tracking, guided resistance are applied to facilitate the movements.

Purpose/Treatment Goals

The purpose is to facilitate the pelvic and lower extremity control needed during forward progression. The procedure is first performed by having the patient move forward and back over one limb. As control is gained, forward progression is allowed. Stance phase control is usually facilitated first followed by control of swing.

Problems with Application

A therapist may apply too much resistance. In this procedure the skill level of control is facilitated in a position where the BoS is very small and the CoG is high. Resistance, therefore, is used only to promote the timing and sequencing of the movement, not to strengthen a muscle or movement. If strengthening is required, a return to less difficult postures, where postural control is less compromised, is necessary. Therapists must observe the entire body movement. Patients may tend to compensate with exaggerated movements in other body parts if ambulation is too challenging. Improper patterns should be discouraged in early stages, otherwise poor habits may develop.

The proper position of the knee is considered. Neither hyperextension nor exaggerated flexion should be allowed. Hyperextension can be caused by limited range of dorsiflexion as well as abnormal strength or tone of the ankle or knee musculature.

During swing the proper sequencing of pelvic and leg movements are emphasized. The pelvis leads the movement with forward rotation and a slight pelvic tilt before the hip and knee are allowed to flex. If pelvic and leg movements occur simultaneously, the leg will tend to circumduct. Conversely, if the leg begins to swing prior to the pelvic movement, the leg may swing through with hip adduction creating a "crab walking" gait pattern. By facilitating the proper timing and sequencing of movement these abnormal patterns can be discouraged.

Some patients may need to simulate the normal speed of gait in addition to focusing on sequencing the components.

Activity: Back walking; side walking

Technique: Resisted progression (RP); MC pelvis

Impairments: Decreased ability to extend the hip and accept weight; decreased lateral pelvic control during weight bearing; weak gluteus maximus or gluteus medius.

66

Description

To resist back walking the therapist may be in front of or behind the patient with MCs on the pelvis. A slight stretch is applied to pelvic rotation to facilitate the pelvic motion and hip extension. To discourage reinforcement of abnormal extensor patterns, hip extension is combined with knee flexion (Fig. 66A).

Side walking may be performed in both directions. The therapist is at the patient's side with one MC on the pelvis and the other on the lateral thigh (Fig. 66B). The abductors of the leading limb swing the leg, a skill level, while the abductors of the stance leg stabilize the body. For patients with movement control deficits, the progression of control is similar to that previously described, beginning with stance and progressing to swing.

Purpose/Treatment Goals

The purposes are to improve the patient's movement in the environment, and promote advanced movement patterns, i.e., hip extension with knee flexion or hip abduction independent of trunk lateral flexion.

Problems with Application

Patients will attempt to perform the procedure with the most readily available pattern which may not be the most desired movement. For example, in side walking the patient may perform

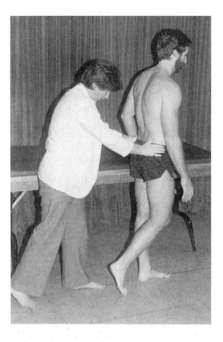

66A Backward walking: Hip extension with knee flexion.

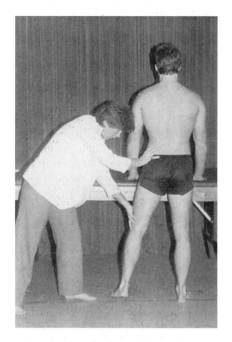

66B Sidewalking: Hip abduction.

hip hiking or may externally rotate and flex the hip to substitute for weakness in the gluteus medius.

67

Activity: Braiding
Technique: SRH; RP; MC pelvis
Impairments: Decreased crossing midline; pelvic rotation.

Description

In this procedure the patient may be at the parallel bars or, if less support is required, at the therapist's side. This is the most difficult of the ambulation activities. The legs cross the midline in diagonal patterns combined with exaggerated lower trunk rotation. One leg crosses in front in the D1F pattern (Fig. 67A); the other moves up and out in D2F. As the legs cross behind, one extends with adduction in D2E (Fig. 67B); the other extends with abduction in D1E. The procedure can be performed in its entirety with the technique of RP or one part can be isolated and emphasized with SRH. For example, the D1F pattern may be emphasized to enhance pelvic forward rotation with hip flexion and adduction. To perform RP, MCs are on the pelvis. A very slight stretch is applied to the pelvic motion followed by tracking resistance to guide the movement.

Purpose/Treatment Goals

The purpose is to (1) combine different patterns of pelvic and hip movement, (2) promote lower trunk rotation in this high level activity, (3) facilitate crossing of the midline, (4) promote postural control responses, (5) emphasize static–dynamic activity in the stance phase limb and (6) enhance inversion–eversion and ankle control.

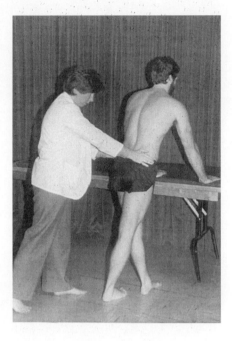

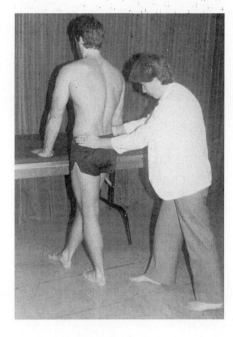

67A Braiding: D1F.

67B Braiding: D2E

Problems with Application

Patients may have difficulty learning the movement combinations. Having the patient mimic the therapist is often successful. To ensure the correct hip rotation during the diagonal patterns, the feet should be in line with the body, pointing straight ahead.

Braiding is the most difficult of the upright sequence procedures and should not be attempted until late in the rehabilitation process. Many other procedures must precede braiding before this high level control can be expected.

Study Questions

1. Compare prone on elbows to quadruped. In your comparison include the following: base of support, center of gravity, the number of weight-bearing joints involved, the length of the lever arm, the effect of placement of manual contacts.

2. Match the following techniques to the stages of control:
   A. Mobility
   B. Stability
   C. Controlled mobility
   D. Skill
   1. Slow reversal hold
   2. Alternating isometrics
   3. Hold relax active motion
   4. Slow reversal
   5. Rhythmic initiation
   6. Shortened held resisted contraction
   7. Resisted progression
   8. Rhythmic stabilization
   9. Agonistic reversals

3. Define dynamic stability. Describe how you would develop it for the upper extremity through a progression of procedures including a sequence of activities and techniques.

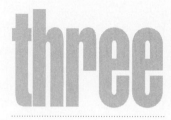

Extremity Procedures

Key Terms

Trunk patterns
Bilateral patterns
Unilateral patterns
Mass pattern
Advanced pattern
Indirect approach
Increments of range
Techniques
Contract relax (CR)
Hold relax (HR)
Normal timing (NT)
Rhythmical rotation (RR)
Timing for emphasis (TE)
Overflow

TRUNK, BILATERAL, UNILATERAL PATTERNS

The extremity patterns can be combined to emphasize the trunk or can be performed in bilateral or unilateral combinations. During the performance of **trunk patterns** the limbs are in contact with each other creating a closed kinematic chain. This body-on-body contact allows the emphasis of the activity to be focused on the trunk. During the trunk patterns the extremities move asymmetrically: one limb moves in the D1 direction and the other in the D2 direction. The body-on-body contact is useful for patients with decreased sensation, neglect of one limb, or the inability to move a limb independently. Because different segments are involved in the trunk patterns, i.e., the head, both upper extremities and the upper trunk, or the lower trunk and both lower extremities, these activities can be used to promote overflow from one body part to another.

Trunk and bilateral patterns focus on proximal muscles.

Bilateral patterns can be performed in one of four combinations.

1. **Symmetrical:** Both limbs move in the same pattern in the same direction, e.g., bilateral symmetrical (BS) D1 flexion
2. **Reciprocal:** Both limbs move in the same pattern but in opposite directions, e.g., bilateral reciprocal (BR) D2; one limb moves in D2F as the other moves in D2E
3. **Asymmetrical:** The limbs move in different diagonals but in the same direction, e.g., bilateral asymmetrical (BA) flexion to the right; the right limb moves in D2F as the left limb moves in D1F
4. **Cross diagonal or reciprocal asymmetrical:** The limbs move in different diagonals in opposite directions, e.g., one limb moves in D2F while the other moves in D1E.

The bilateral combinations similar to the trunk patterns can be performed to facilitate trunk activity or to promote overflow from one limb to the other. The focus of the patterns is primarily proximal, i.e., the scapula and the shoulder or the pelvis and the hip. The intermediate joint, the elbow or the knee, usually remains straight.

Unilateral patterns focus on proximal, intermediate and distal muscles.

Unilateral patterns can be performed with the intermediate joint in different positions:

1. Straight throughout the movement
2. Flexing or extending during proximal joint flexion or extension, respectively termed a mass flexion or extension motion in the LE
3. Extending during proximal joint flexion or flexing during proximal joint extension termed an advanced combination of the lower extremity.

Both of the therapist's MCs are on one limb during the performance of unilateral patterns, giving the therapist the best control of the limb movement.

In treatment, the sequence of procedures usually progresses from trunk to bilateral to unilateral combinations. This sequence proceeds from the easiest to the most difficult for an individual limb to perform. Specific indications for each individual procedure or pattern are included with the description of the procedure.

The stages of control that can best be promoted with these patterns are **mobility,** either ROM or initiation of movement, **stability** or **skill,** the normal timing of movement. Strengthening procedures can be performed at all stages.

Upper Trunk

Activity: Supine; upper trunk flexion (Chop)
Technique: Slow reversal hold (SRH); MC on head and wrist.
Impairments: Weak abdominals; restricted trunk rotation; decreased interaction of left and right sides of body; weakness in one upper extremity or pain and extreme weakness or muscle inhibition in lower extremities.

68

Chop combines bilateral upper extremity extension with trunk flexion.

Description

This activity can be performed either to the right or the left. In this sequence trunk flexion or a chop to the *right* is described. The therapist positions the patient near the edge of the plinth so that the patient can be adequately guided and resisted throughout the movement. The therapist is positioned at the patient's side. This procedure combines the upper extremities in an asymmetrical pattern with body-on-body contact. The patient's right, or lead, arm moves in the D1 pattern; the left, or assisting, arm moves in D2. The patient's D2 (left) hand grasps the forearm of the D1 arm. The right hand of the therapist is on the patient's right wrist and the therapist's left hand on the crown of the head. To teach the patient the movement, the therapist passively flexes the patient's arms up and across the face and extends the head into the reverse direction or reverse chop. The therapist then changes direction into the trunk flexion movement, i.e., the head is flexed with rotation and the limbs are extended to the right. The movement occurs in a diagonal but straight line. Circular movements overemphasizing shoulder abduction or adduction should be avoided.

To resist the movement, the patient is positioned in the lengthened range of the chop (reverse chop—the arms up and across the face) (Fig. 68A). The chopping motion is facilitated by a quick stretch applied to the limbs into the direction of flexion, adduction (of the leading UE), and rotation, and is combined with a traction force. Little or no stretch is applied to the head. When the stretch is applied to the UEs, the abdominal muscles, which will flex and rotate the upper trunk, are simultaneously stretched. Following the quick stretch, resistance is provided to the movement of the arms extending down and across the body, the head, and the upper trunk flexion with rotation. When the patient reaches the shortened range of the chop all components of the pattern are isometrically resisted and further facilitated by an approximation force. Resistance in this shortened range is applied in the direction of the opposite shoulder (Fig. 68B). Quick stretch and resistance is then applied to the antagonistic movement of trunk extension with rotation and UE flexion, i.e., the reverse chop. Verbal commands might be "bring your arms down to your side and flex your head and curl your upper body (chop), hold it there, now bring your arms up and across your face, keep your eyes on your hand and extend your head" (reverse chop) (Figs. 68C, 68D). The series of slow reversals begins with a small amount of resistance that increases with each reversal. Because the neck flexors are not very strong, resistance to the head during the chopping motion is minimal. By maintaining the MCs on the crown of the head either assistance or resistance can be provided. The head and the UEs act as one unit to promote the trunk motion.

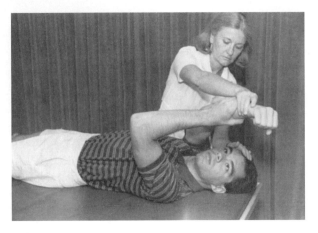

68A Chop—lengthened range.

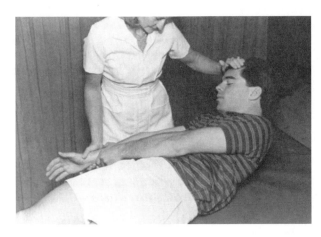

68B Chop—shortened range.

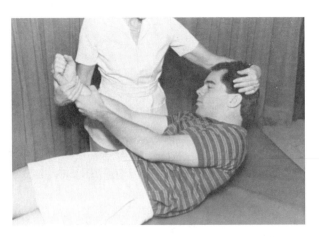

68C Reverse chop—lengthened range.

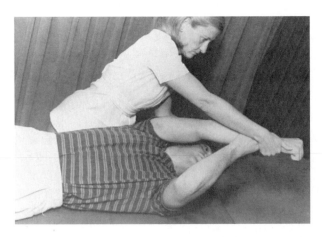

68D Reverse chop—shortened range.

Purpose/Treatment Goals

The purposes are to promote trunk flexion with rotation; to strengthen the abdominals, primarily the upper abdominals; to enhance crossing of the midline to promote an interaction between the two sides of the body; to facilitate rolling; to promote overflow from one UE to the other and to the lower extremities; and to facilitate a reversal of antagonists.

The trunk muscles that are primarily active in the chop to the right are the left upper abdominal and the right lower abdominals. During the chopping motion and especially with the hold in the shortened range of the chop, overflow to the lower extremities may be noted.

For patients with paraparesis, rolling is facilitated in the direction of the chop and the UEs can be used to enhance the momentum of the rolling motion.

Hemiparetic patients who demonstrate a unilateral deficit may find rolling toward the uninvolved side in the direction of the reverse chop easier. In addition, the involved UE moves in D1F (flexion with adduction), which is out of synergistic movements.

Problems with Application

The therapist should be properly positioned in the diagonal pattern to best facilitate the patient's movement.

The MC on the wrist provides the resistance to the limbs for purposes of emphasizing the trunk pattern, not just the extremity motions. In the shortened range of the chop, the therapist may incorrectly overemphasize resistance to the lead arm (in D1E) rather than resisting the trunk motion of flexion with rotation. Trunk resistance is directed toward the opposite shoulder.

When the chop is performed in this supine position the trunk is flexing against gravity as well as manual resistance. Care must be taken therefore not to overpower the patient.

The therapist has a tendency to apply too much resistance as the patient initiates the chopping motion when the arms are up across the face and just beginning to extend. Too much resistance to the isotonic motion in the lengthened range and during the entire movement will cause the patient to move in a circular direction and "windmill" rather than stay in the diagonal or the "groove" of the pattern. The therapist needs to guide the patient into the correct motion.

Chop facilitates primarily upper abdominal and upper extremity muscles of the D1, D2 extensor patterns.

Activity: Supine; upper trunk flexion (chop)
Technique: Slow reversal hold (SRH) with timing for emphasis (TE); MC on head and wrist.
Impairments: Weak upper abdominals; weakness in muscles of extremity extensor patterns; decreased interaction of both sides of the body; extreme muscle weakness or inhibition of lower extremities.

69

TE to chop will facilitate quadriceps contraction.

Description

The activity of upper trunk flexion, chopping, is the same as that previously described. The purpose of the technique of timing for emphasis is to strengthen specific muscles within a pattern and is indicated when an imbalance of strength exists, i.e., some muscles are stronger than others in the pattern. In this procedure the assumption is made that the patient has stronger muscles in the neck and the arms than in the trunk, for example, a paraparetic patient with a lesion at T10. The stronger muscles of the head, neck, and UEs are resisted into the range in which they can hold best. An isometric contraction to promote overflow into the weaker abdominal muscles is then applied. As a general rule, extensor muscles hold best near their shortened range and flexors at approximately 90 degrees. In this example, the isometric hold is performed with the neck and shoulders in the shortened range of the chop. In this shortened range the stronger components, the head and the arms, are "locked in," which means that a strong isometric contraction facilitated by approximation is performed. The weaker abdominal muscles are then "pivoted" or facilitated by stretch and isotonic resistance, i.e., repeated contractions.

The entire procedure is as follows. At the beginning of the procedure, the technique of SRH is repeated a few times to ensure that both the therapist and the patient are performing the movement correctly. The technique of TE is then performed by first resisting the head and the extremities into their shortened ranges where an isometric contraction of these segments is resisted. While maintaining resistance to these stronger parts, a quick stretch to the trunk muscles is applied by approximating the arms and the head in a diagonal direction back toward the opposite shoulder. Because the arms are "locked in," the stretch actually occurs in the trunk muscles. The trunk is then resisted but allowed to continue to flex and rotate. When the patient's effort diminishes, the stretch is reapplied to the contracting trunk muscles and the subsequent movement resisted again. The patient may need to perform a series of three or four of these repeated contractions to complete the movement into the shortened range of trunk flexion with rotation. The patient's head and UE remain in relatively the same position as the trunk continues to flex and rotate. Remember, however, that because the patient is flexing against gravity, the manual resistance provided should facilitate and not overcome the contraction. After the last repeated contraction or pivot to the abdominals, an isometric hold is applied to all components in the shortened range of the pattern and the reversal movement, reverse chop, is facilitated by a stretch.

Timing for emphasis elicits irradiation effects from strong to weak muscles.

Verbal commands may be "bring your arms and head down to the side" (isotonic resistance to the stronger parts through range), "now hold them there" (isometric resistance to lock in the stronger segments), "curl your trunk" or "lift your opposite shoulder off the plinth and keep moving" (repeated contractions to the trunk flexors), "now hold the entire pattern" (isometric contraction), and lastly, "move your arms up and across your face" (the reversal movement is stretched and resisted).

Purpose/Treatment Goals

The purposes are to strengthen the upper abdominals by facilitating overflow from the stronger upper body segments and to provide overflow to lower extremities.

The reversal motion is performed to facilitate the chop via successive induction and to reduce fatigue caused by continuous contraction in the muscles to be strengthened. Successive induction means the facilitation of a muscle or movement pattern by previously performing the antagonistic movement or pattern.

Problems with Application

Therapists have a tendency to perform the repeated contractions to the abdominals in a small portion of the range rather than allowing the patient to move through the complete range, to apply too much resistance following the quick stretch and overcome the patient's effort, or to assist the patient with the movement. Providing the appropriate amount of resistance that will facilitate the contraction through range is difficult. Included in this manual are other examples of TE so therapists will have ample opportunity to practice this very useful strengthening technique.

Because maximum effort is desired with the technique of TE, only a few repetitions of the technique are appropriate.

Therapists may not adequately "lock in" the stronger parts and may incorrectly rush into the repeated contractions of the weaker muscles. The patient must be given sufficient time to develop a maximum isometric contraction to ensure that overflow from the stronger to the weaker muscles occurs. The amount of time needed depends on the strength of the patient and the skill of the therapist. Adding approximation may help to promote this isometric contraction.

Activity: Supine; chop and reverse chop
Technique: Slow reversal hold (SRH); contacts on scapula
Impairments: Weak scapular protraction and retraction; decreased scapulohumeral rhythm; dominance of synergistic activity.

70

Manual contacts are positioned proximally for increased scapular control.

Description

The activity performed by the patient is the same as in the previous procedures only now the focus is on scapula motion. When one specific part of the pattern is emphasized, control over other aspects of the pattern is sacrificed. In this procedure the patient has to be able to perform the pattern as active motion without the assistance of the therapist's MCs.

To ensure that the correct pattern is performed, the patient is first guided through the movement. To emphasize the scapula movement during the reverse chop motion, both MCs with fingers interdigitated or overlapping are placed over the proximal anterior shoulder region. If the fingertips are just touching, there is a tendency to "dig in" with the fingers. One MC is between the patient's arm and body and one lateral to the patient's arm. The scapula motion that is promoted during the reverse chop is protraction. To perform the chop and promote scapula retraction, the therapist's hands are moved to the dorsal medial surface of the scapula. The lateral hand is moved first to initially resist the movement, then the other MC is placed under the scapula. With verbal cues the therapist guides the movement of the patient's UE onto the therapist's shoulder. The therapist can resist the patient's extremity movements although the major focus remains proximal.

Purpose/Treatment Goals

The purposes are to facilitate scapula motion and promote scapulohumeral rhythm and promote movement out of synergy.

In addition to the technique of SRH, RC can be used to emphasize the proximal muscles. The serratus anterior is the prime mover as the lead UE moves into D1F during the reverse chop and the rhomboids are facilitated as the D1E pattern is performed during the chop.

Problems with Application

The therapist may have difficulty positioning MCs and moving them during the reversals. The lateral MC moves first and is followed by the MC between the patient's arm and body.

71

*Reverse chop promotes
shoulder mobility in
the D1 direction.*

Activity: Supine; reverse chop
Technique: Hold relax (HR) or rhythmic stabilization (RS); MC on fore-arms
Impairments: Tightness of shoulder extensors or internal rotators; shoulder pain; decreased scapular stability.

Description

HR and RS are used to gain ROM by increasing the extensibility of the contractile tissues. The extremity motions that occur during the trunk pattern are the focus of the procedure, in contrast with the previous procedures that emphasized the trunk muscles. The body-on-body contact, which occurs in this trunk pattern will allow the patient to control and assist the movement of an involved, painful, or weak extremity.

The therapist stands at the patient's side in the direction of the diagonal pattern or at the patient's head to emphasize the shortened range. With the therapist's MCs on the patient's fore-arms, the patient flexes the limbs up and across the face, in the reverse chop, to the point of range limitation. The involved UE moves in the D1F pattern; HR is then applied. The isometric contraction can be applied either to the agonists (the muscles that move the limb into the desired range) (Fig. 71A), or the antagonists (the range limiting muscles) (Fig. 71B). HR involves a slow buildup of isometric force until a moderate contraction is achieved. Slow relaxation of the contraction is followed by active movement with tracking resistance into the new range. The verbal commands are "hold, relax, now move up and across your face." The technique is reapplied until no additional range is achieved. To be effective the technique must incorporate a slow buildup of resistance, supportive but gentle MCs, and calm, soothing verbal commands. The active movement promotes muscular contraction of the agonist into the new range and reciprocal inhibition of the antagonist.

RS also can be used to increase range. In previous procedures RS has been used to promote stability. To gain range or increase mobility the technique is applied in a slightly different manner. With the therapist's MCs on the forearms, the patient moves into the reverse chop with minimal resistance to the point of limitation. In this range an isometric hold is applied to the agonist. Without allowing any relaxation to occur the therapist changes the resistive force of one MC to the other direction so that resistance is simultaneously applied to the antagonist of one limb and the agonist of the other (Fig. 71C). Resistance is thus applied to the two limbs in oppo-

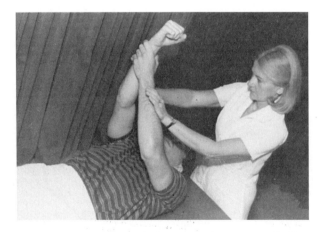

71A Reverse chop—HR to agonists.

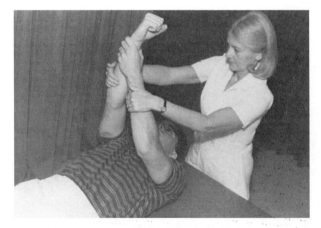

71B Reverse chop—HR to antagonists.

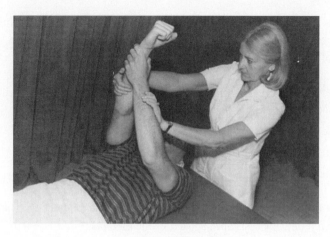

71C Reverse chop—RS.

site directions at the same time. One limb is holding with flexors, the other with extensors. The resistive force of both MCs is then reversed simultaneously and the isometric contraction gradually increased. This change of resistance is repeated a few times. Isometric resistance is finally applied with both MCs to the agonist (flexors) followed by a slightly resisted movement into more flexion. When the new range has been gained, the cycle of isometric contractions is repeated: isometric resistance in opposite directions, then resistance to the agonist and isotonic movement into the new range.

If elbow extension, rather than shoulder flexion, is limited, both MCs can be placed on the involved arm above and below the elbow. Either of these two techniques, HR or RS, can be performed. When movement into elbow extension is desired the triceps are the agonistic muscle group. To perform these techniques on the elbow, the shoulders are maintained between 60 and 90 degrees of flexion and the elbow moved into the shortened range of extension. The isometric contraction to the elbow extensors is emphasized during this mobility procedure, both to enhance the triceps response and to reciprocally inhibit the elbow flexors. If, in contrast, elbow flexion is limited, the technique is performed with the flexors acting as the agonists.

Purpose/Treatment Goals

The purpose is to increase **mobility,** ROM into shoulder flexion, adduction, and external rotation, or into elbow extension by increasing the extensibility of the contractile tissues.

These relaxation techniques are designed to affect the contractile tissues. Joint mobilization procedures to increase the extensibility of the noncontractile tissues may need to accompany the exercise procedures to ensure that complete range is gained.

HR performed to the agonist is a preferred technique. When applied in this manner an isometric contraction of the agonist and reciprocal inhibition of the antagonist occur simultaneously. In addition, the therapist's resistance is into the pain-free range, which may elicit more cooperation from the patient. If the limb is painful, the therapist must allow the patient to relax slowly as quick relaxation can elicit pain.

The technique of RS, although slightly more difficult to perform than HR, is extremely effective for patients who exhibit muscle splinting because of pain, e.g., burn patients. In these cases range may be limited by tightness of the skin as well as of the contractile tissue. Increases in range which result from this technique may be due to the slight shearing force that occurs between the muscle and the overlying skin during the intermittent muscular contraction and relaxation.

Isometric techniques are used to promote mobility when pain is a factor.

For patients with poor proximal stability and who cannot tolerate weight-bearing postures, i.e., post-upper extremity fractures, the technique of RS can be performed to improve the stability functioning of the scapula and the shoulder muscles.

Isometric contractions of the muscles of the hand and the wrist also occur during the performance of these techniques. Both HR and RS applied in the manner described can be used as an indirect approach in cases of distal involvement.

Problems with Application

The therapist may elicit an isometric "push" rather than an isometric "hold" by incorrectly asking the patient to pull the arm up and across during the holding contractions. A "hold" command will allow the therapist to control the magnitude of the contraction. The patient should match and not overcome the resistance applied by the therapist.

As mentioned, slow relaxation of the contraction is important if the patient is in pain. An increase in involuntary holding, or splinting, may result if the contraction is relaxed too quickly.

In both techniques, active movement into the new range will perpetuate the contraction of the agonist and the inhibition to the antagonist as well as reduce the pain and apprehension often associated with passive stretching.

72

Activity: Supine; upper trunk extension (Lift)

Technique: Slow reversal hold (SRH) with timing for emphasis (TE); MC head and wrist

Impairments: Weak upper trunk extensors; weakness in muscles of extremity flexor patterns; decreased interaction of both sides of the body; restricted trunk rotation

Lift combines bilateral upper extremity flexion with trunk extension.

Description

Trunk extension with rotation occurs in the lifting motion as the extremities move in asymmetrical flexion patterns. During lifting to the *right* the patient's right arm leads the movement in D2F; the left arm is in D1F and assists by holding on at the right forearm or wrists.

The therapist stands at the head of the plinth in the diagonal direction. To ensure neck and trunk extension, the patient's head should be off the plinth but supported by the therapist at all times. The therapist positions one MC on the patient's right wrist and the other on the patient's head. The activity begins in the lengthened range of the lift with the arms in extension across the opposite hip; the head is flexed and rotated to the left. To teach the patient the movement pattern, the arms are guided into shoulder flexion with the lead arm abducting (D2F) while the head extends. The patient is instructed to watch the hands to promote head participation in the movement.

Once the patient is familiar with the movement, the pattern can be resisted. Movement is facilitated with a quick stretch in the lengthened range of the lift (Fig. 72A). The stretch is primarily a traction and rotation force applied to the upper trunk and limbs; no stretch is applied to the head and the neck. The lift is resisted into the shortened range where an isometric hold is performed (Fig. 72B). To facilitate the hold the therapist can add either a traction or an approximation force depending on the patient's response. A quick stretch is then applied to facilitate the antagonistic movement. The quick stretch in this range of shoulder flexion should only be a traction, rotational force and *not* movement into more shoulder flexion. Following the stretch, the movement into the reverse lift is resisted and an isometric hold with approximation is applied in the shortened range. One MC stays on the crown of the head and pivots around the

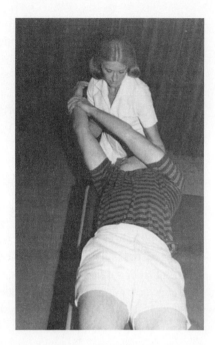

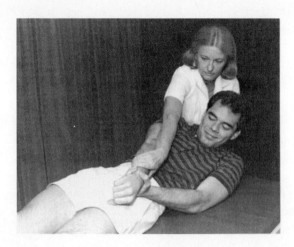

72A Lift—lengthened range.   **72B** Lift—shortened range.

head from forearm pronation when resisting head flexion, to supination when resisting head extension. Both excessive resistance to neck flexion and movement into extreme neck extension are avoided.

If the patient's arms are stronger than the upper trunk, the technique of TE is indicated to strengthen the weaker upper trunk extensors. To perform TE, the stronger UEs are resisted into the shortened range of flexion where an isometric contraction of the lifting pattern is performed. The head and arms are "locked in" with a traction or approximation force. Repeated contractions are then applied to the back extensors to facilitate movement into trunk extension with rotation. When the shortened range is achieved, an isometric contraction of the entire pattern is resisted, followed by facilitation of the reversal pattern.

Purpose/Treatment Goals

The purposes are to strengthen upper trunk extension with rotation; to enhance movement of the lead UE into the D2F pattern; to promote overflow from the UEs into the trunk and LEs; and to promote interaction of both sides of the body.

In this activity the back extensors are assisted by gravity, therefore the therapist must provide sufficient resistance to the movement, which may be difficult with a large patient. When the upper back extensors have gained sufficient strength to overcome gravity, a more challenging position, such as sitting or prone, is indicated.

Problems with Application

The therapist needs to be positioned properly and move in the diagonal direction with the patient. As the UEs near the shortened range of the lift, the therapist needs to bend at the knees to adequately resist the movement. Some therapists may find practicing TE to the lift in supine too difficult if the partner is large and of normal strength. However, patients with trunk extensor strength below a fair grade may benefit from this gravity-assisted position.

Stretch to the reverse lift is primarily a traction force. Attempting to move into more shoul-

Lift facilitates primarily upper trunk extensors and muscles of the D1, D2 flexor patterns.

der flexion, abduction, and external rotation would create an anterior dislocating force on the glenohumeral joint and should be avoided.

73

Activity: Supine; trunk extension (lift)

Technique: Hold relax (HR) or rhythmic stabilization (RS); MC on forearms

Impairments: Tightness of shoulder extensors or internal rotators; shoulder pain; decreased scapular stability.

Lift promotes shoulder mobility in the D2 direction.

Description

This procedure can promote an increase in ROM into shoulder flexion, abduction and external rotation, D2F. Similar to the reverse chop, assistance is provided by the intact UE. The techniques of HR and RS can be applied in this pattern in the same manner as previously described for the reverse chop. The lift or shoulder flexion with abduction is the agonistic motion; the reverse lift or shoulder extension with adduction is the range limiting, antagonistic pattern.

The therapist is positioned at the head of the plinth in the diagonal of the pattern. Because the goal is to increase the range of shoulder motion, MCs can be placed on both forearms or both MCs can be placed on the lead UE. To briefly review the techniques, the arms are minimally resisted to the point of limitation where a slow buildup of isometric resistance to the agonists is given. With the technique of HR, the isometric contraction is followed by slow relaxation and then active movement into the new range (Fig. 73A). Verbal commands are "hold, relax, now move your arms over your head." The isometric resistance also can be applied to the antagonistic muscle groups followed by active movement into the agonistic range.

To perform RS to increase ROM, the pattern is resisted to the point of limitation. At this range an isometric contraction of the agonists is followed by simultaneous resistance in opposite directions, which is reversed and repeated a few times (Fig. 73B). Resistance to the agonist

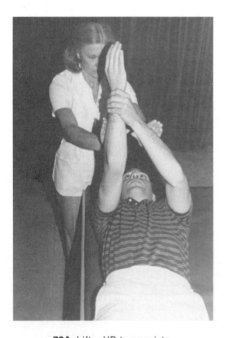

73A Lift—HR to agonists.

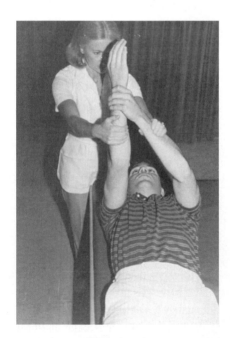

73B Lift—RS.

with both MCs occurs again followed by isotonic resistance into the new range. The sequence continues until no additional range is gained (Review Procedure 71).

Purpose/Treatment Goals

The purpose is to increase mobility, i.e., ROM into shoulder flexion, abduction, and external rotation (D2F).

The combination of movements that occurs in D2F are the same as the limitations which occur in the capsular pattern of the shoulder: flexion, abduction, and external rotation. Movement in the D1 pattern (reverse chop) is usually less painful and difficult for the patient and should precede movement into D2F in a treatment progression. In addition to these techniques to increase the length of the contractile tissues, joint mobilization procedures and thermal modalities may be used to increase the extensibility of the noncontractile tissues. Following the gains in range or mobility, the next stage of control, i.e., stability, can be incorporated into the treatment.

HR and RS can also be performed to the lift in a sitting position. Because the scapular movement is not restricted by the plinth, scapula elevation may be more easily achieved in this posture.

Stability of the scapula is dependent on many factors, including control in the middle and the lower trapezius. The trapezius is the scapular muscle primarily active in the D2F pattern. RS applied to the lift in either supine or sitting may achieve the important goal of increased scapular stability.

Shoulder flexion range in the D2 direction is greater than in the D1 direction.

Problems with Application

Therapists may give too much resistance or move the patient too quickly into new ranges. To accomplish the goals of muscle relaxation and movement without pain, the therapist must be sensitive to the patient's responses.

Upper trunk patterns can be performed independently as active movement or with weights.

SUMMARY—UPPER TRUNK PROCEDURES

Trunk patterns can be incorporated into the treatment for purposes other than those described. The reverse chop can promote rolling from supine toward prone and is particularly beneficial for those patients with unilateral neglect or inability to move one limb. Rolling to supine, although not as frequent a problem, can be promoted with a lift. An alternative to these trunk patterns is to have the patient grasp the two hands together in a prayer position to assist rolling. The trunk patterns can be performed in sitting to strengthen or promote stability in the trunk, UE musculature, or to challenge sitting balance. The chop can assist with the initial phase and the lift, the final phase of the assumption of kneeling. Both trunk patterns facilitate overflow to the lower extremities and therefore can be an indirect method of activating LE musculature. To improve ROM at the scapula or shoulder, the patient may cradle the involved arm at the elbow, which will reduce the length of the lever arm and lessen the difficulty of the procedure. Lastly, these patterns are easily incorporated into home programs and can be performed as either active or resistive movement.

Bilateral Upper Extremity

The trunk flexion and extension patterns that may precede these bilateral and unilateral patterns during treatment have been described. The bilateral patterns can be performed in four combinations, symmetrical, reciprocal, asymmetrical, and cross diagonal. The unilateral patterns can be performed with the elbow straight, flexing, or extending throughout the movement. The therapist chooses the appropriate combinations based on impairments and the goals of the procedure, the patient's pattern of reinforcement (symmetrical or reciprocal), and the pattern of strength.

74

Activity: Supine; bilateral symmetrical diagonal 2 flexion (BS D2F)
Technique: Slow reversal hold (SRH) with rhythmic stabilization (RS) and timing for emphasis (TE); MC on wrists
Impairments: Difficulty reversing movements in a coordinated manner; decreased scapular or upper trunk stability; bilateral or unilateral shoulder weakness.

Description

The patient is positioned near the top edge of the plinth and the therapist stands at the patient's head. The therapist's feet are positioned one in front of the other to allow the therapist movement in a forward and backward direction as the patient flexes and extends the UEs.

To begin, the patient's arms are crossed over the body with thumbs on opposite hips in D2E. The therapist's MCs are on the patient's wrists or distal forearms as the patient's UEs are guided through the pattern. The pattern is then resisted beginning in the lengthened range of D2F (Fig. 74A). The stretch to facilitate the pattern is largely a traction, rotatory force. The distal component of wrist and finger extension with forearm supination leads the movement as the therapist resists the arms into the shortened range of D2F where an isometric contraction is performed (Fig. 74B). To facilitate the hold either a traction or an approximation force may be used. To initiate movement into the antagonist D2E pattern a traction, rotatory stretch is applied to the muscles performing D2E (Fig. 74C). The therapist must be careful not to overstretch the anterior capsule of the shoulder in this position. Following this stretch, resistance is applied to the D2E pattern and the hold in the shortened range is enhanced with approximation. Throughout each direction of movement the therapist must allow rotation of the patient's forearm and shoulder to occur. MCs, therefore, cannot be too firm.

A patient may demonstrate functional limitations and have difficulty with smooth coordinated UE movement at approximately 90 degrees of shoulder flexion due to the long lever arm

Many techniques can be combined with bilateral or reciprocal patterns to promote movement control or strength.

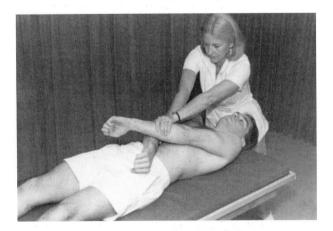

74A BS D2F—lengthened range.

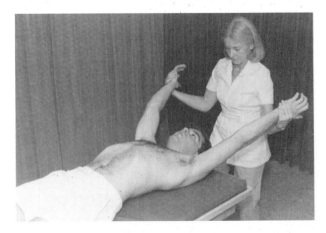

74B BS D2F—shortened range.

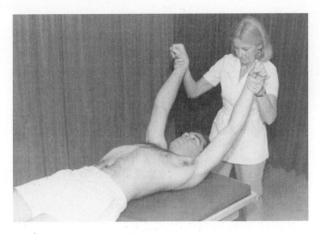

74C BS D2E—lengthened range.

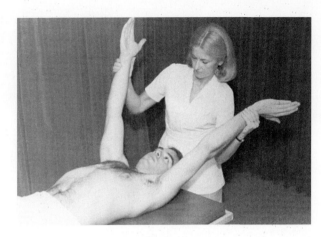

74D BS D2F—TE to LUE

that exists in this range. The deficit may be poor dynamic stability of the proximal muscles. Improved stability in the proximal scapula and shoulder may be promoted by the technique of RS performed at the 90-degree range. To perform this procedure the bilateral D2F pattern is resisted to 90 degrees, where RS is applied. RS begins with isometric resistance simultaneously applied to both UEs in D2F. The resistance applied by one MC is altered to the other side of one forearm and resistance is applied to that limb in the D2E pattern as the other is resisted in D2F, i.e., they are holding in a reciprocal combination. After a buildup of isometric tension has been achieved the therapist gradually and simultaneously switches resistance to the opposite direction by changing pressure to the other side of the forearm. This reversal of isometric resistance is continued for a few repetitions until a strong holding contraction occurs. The last hold is applied to the symmetrical D2F pattern followed by isotonic resistance throughout the rest of the range.

Some patients can reinforce best in the reciprocal manner described whereas others seem unstable and have difficulty coordinating smooth isometric reversals. In such cases the technique of AI, in which alternating isometric resistance is applied symmetrically in the D2 pattern, may be more beneficial.

TE is an appropriate technique when one UE is weaker than the other and the goal of the procedure is to strengthen the proximal components of one limb. TE to D2F is begun in the lengthened range of the pattern by positioning the stronger limb over the weaker so the patient can lead from strength. Both UEs are stretched and resisted into D2F. When the stronger limb reaches 90 degrees, it is locked in with an isometric contraction. The weaker limb is then pivoted throughout the range of D2F (Fig. 74D) and isometrically resisted in the shortened range. Both limbs are then reversed into D2E. The stronger arm, which has been holding at 90 degrees, can reverse direction from that angle.

TE can be combined with the RS or AI techniques. For example, after a few repetitions of isometric holding at 90 degrees (AI or RS), isometric resistance is maintained on the stronger limb while the other limb is pivoted further into D2F.

TE can be similarly performed to D2E when the goal is strengthening the sternal portion of the pectoralis major. While moving into D2E, the stronger limb is isometrically resisted at 90 to 70 degrees and the weaker limb pivoted into D2E (Fig. 74E).

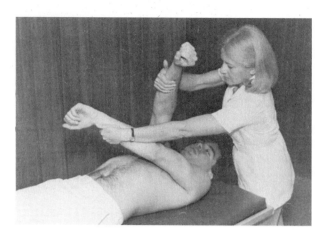

74E BS D2E—TE to LUE

Purpose/Treatment Goals

The purposes are to promote a smooth reversal of antagonistic muscles (SRH); to enhance stability of the shoulder and upper trunk (AI or RS); and to strengthen the trapezius and middle deltoid in D2F and the pectoralis minor and sternal portion of the pectoralis major in D2E (TE).

Breathing patterns can be easily incorporated into these motions: inspiration with D2F and expiration with D2E. The symmetrical extremity patterns also enhance trunk flexion or extension.

RS applied to the upper extremities in the manner described can be used to activate the rotator cuff muscles and improve the position of the humeral head in the glenoid fossa. It can also be used as an indirect approach to facilitate contraction of the trunk muscles. Approximation may be applied to facilitate holding at 90 degrees or in the shortened range of D2F.

The goal of improving dynamic stability in the proximal scapular and shoulder muscles also can be achieved in weight-bearing activities.

Problems with Application

The therapists may hold onto the wrists too tightly and limit rotation of the shoulder and the forearm. Although resisting rotation is important, the therapist should not prevent the motion from occurring.

If the therapist does not move forward and backward with the movement, the patient's arm motion may be limited. In addition, shoulder horizontal abduction-adduction will be overemphasized and the limb movement will not be performed in the proper diagonal groove of the pattern.

Activity: Supine; bilateral reciprocal, BR D2

Technique: Slow reversal hold (SRH) with timing for emphasis (TE) and rhythmic stabilization (RS); MC on wrists

Impairments: Difficulty reversing movements; weakness in bilateral or unilateral proximal shoulder muscles; decreased proximal stability; decreased upper trunk rotation.

75

Description

During bilateral reciprocal D2, one arm moves into the flexion pattern (D2F) while the other moves into extension (D2E). The patient and the MCs are in the same position as described in the preceding procedure. The patient's UEs are first moved symmetrically to familiarize the patient with the pattern. One arm is reversed into the opposite direction and both arms are guided into the reciprocal pattern, one moving in D2F and the other in D2E (Figs. 75A, 75B). The therapist's LE must move with the patient's movement, i.e., as one arm is in extension, the same foot of the therapist is forward and moves back as the patient's arm flexes. The verbal commands are simply "change" or "switch" rather than attempting to give specific instructions pertaining to each part of the pattern.

As with the symmetrical pattern, other techniques can be added such as TE and RS. In TE, where the goal is to improve strength of specific muscle groups, the patient is reinforcing with overflow from reciprocal muscles. For example, a strong middle deltoid on one limb can be used for overflow to a weak sternal portion of the pectoralis major on the opposite side. RS, to improve proximal stability, is performed in a similar manner to that described with the symmetrical combination.

Purpose/Treatment Goals

The purposes are to (1) enhance reciprocal movements in the upper extremities (SRH or SR), (2) strengthen one limb by promoting overflow from the other (TE), (3) promote proximal strength and stability of shoulders and trunk (RS), and (4) facilitate upper trunk rotation and the reciprocal limb movements.

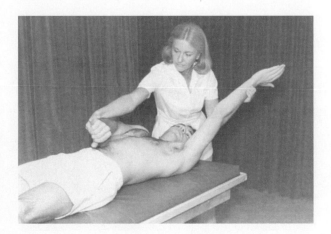

75A Reciprocal D2.

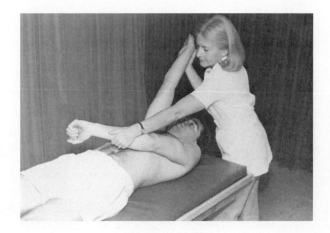

75B Reciprocal D2.

This reciprocal pattern is preferred if the patient reinforces better with a reciprocal rather than a bilateral combination.

Problems with Application

As with the preceding procedure, therapists will tend to hold onto the patient's wrists or forearms too tightly and limit rotational movement. Circular "windmilling" extremity motions may result. If the patient's arms are long, the therapist may need either to move MCs more proximally or to limit the range through which the patient moves.

76

Activity: Supine; bilateral asymmetrical, BA

Technique: Slow reversal hold (SRH) with timing for emphasis (TE); MC on wrists or forearms

Impairments: Difficulty reversing movements; unilateral weakness; decreased trunk rotation.

Description

The asymmetrical patterns combine D1F of one limb with D2F of the other. This combination is most appropriate, for example, when the patient's pattern of strength is such that the middle deltoid can provide overflow to the contralateral anterior deltoid or the sternal pectoralis major can reinforce the activity of the contralateral posterior deltoid. The therapist is positioned at the head of the patient in the diagonal direction of the pattern to emphasize the shoulder flexion motion. With MCs on the wrists or forearms the therapist guides the patient through the pattern: one arm moves in D1 and the other in D2 (Fig. 76A). The verbal commands are "bring your hands up and over to the left and down to the right." With the therapist positioned at the head of the plinth to emphasize shoulder flexion, control and range into the shortened range of extension may be limited (Fig. 76B). TE may be applied in this pattern, e.g., the stronger middle deltoid (D2F) of one limb can be locked in and the opposite weaker anterior deltoid (D1F) pivoted (Fig. 76C). In the extension patterns TE could be used with a strong posterior deltoid

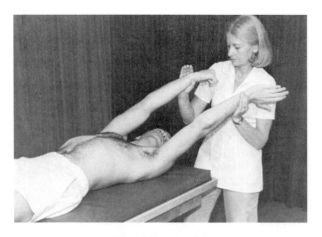

76A BA flexion to left.

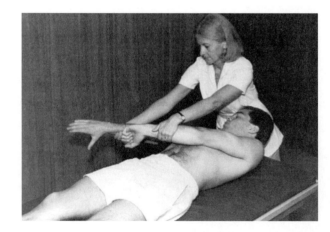

76B BA extension to right.

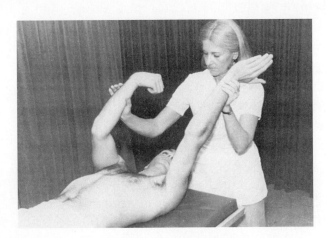

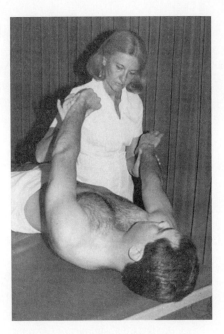

76C BA flexion to left—TE D1F.

76D BA extension to right—TE D2E.

(D1E) to reinforce a weaker sternal portion of the pectoralis major (D2E) (Fig. 76D). The therapist may be positioned by the patient's hip if the emphasis is on extension.

Purpose/Treatment Goals

The purposes are to (1) promote asymmetrical patterns, (2) enhance a smooth reversal of antagonists (SR), (3) enhance overflow from one limb to the other (TE), and (4) promote trunk rotation.

Problems with Application

If the therapist is not positioned in the diagonal direction of the pattern, the movement will not be correct and usually the adduction-abduction components will be overemphasized. If the focus of the procedure is to improve proximal control, less attention may be given to specific distal movements.

Therapists frequently have difficulty controlling or guiding the proper rotational movements of the shoulder: both limbs are externally rotating with shoulder flexion and internally rotating with extension. Performing the patterns slowly will help ensure the proper diagonal direction of the pattern.

77

Activity: Supine; cross diagonal; or reciprocal asymmetrical

Technique: Slow reversal (SR), rhythmic stabilization (RS), timing for emphasis (TE); MC on distal forearms

Impairments: Decreased proximal stability; decreased coordination of movements; unilateral weakness.

Description

In this procedure the extremities move in the two diagonals in opposite directions. The therapist begins by guiding the arms in the asymmetrical combination. One arm is then reversed so that the patient is performing reciprocal asymmetrical movements or the cross-diagonal pattern. Verbal commands may be "open your hands and move your arms apart, now fist your hands and cross your arms" (Fig. 77A).

Purpose/Treatment Goals

The purpose is to strengthen shoulder and trunk (SR); to strengthen proximal scapula and shoulder muscles by promoting overflow from the stronger contralateral limb (TE); to promote proximal stability of the upper trunk and upper extremities (RS).

Because the arms are moving in opposite directions simultaneously both trunk flexors and extensors are facilitated enhancing proximal stability. The applications of RS can further enhance this stability.

The MCs for all of the previously described bilateral patterns were on the wrists or distal forearms. For some patients, especially quadriplegic, MCs may have to be moved more proximally to the elbows to adequately resist the scapular and shoulder muscles.

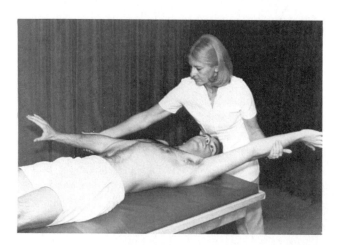

77A Cross diagonal or reciprocal asymmetrical.

Activity: Supine; BS D1 thrust

Technique: Slow reversal hold (SRH) with timing for emphasis (TE); MC on hands

Impairments: Weakness in scapular, shoulder, elbow or finger muscles; movement in synergistic patterns.

78

Description

The therapist stands at the head of the plinth with one leg in front of the other facing the patient. The patient's UEs are positioned in the D1 withdrawal pattern combining shoulder extension, abduction, internal rotation, elbow flexion, forearm supination, wrist flexion with radial deviation, and finger flexion. The fisted hands are anterior to the shoulders.

The therapist's arms are crossed and MCs placed on the extensor surface of the patient's wrists (Fig. 78A). The patient's arms are guided up and across the face into D1 thrust, which combines shoulder flexion, adduction, external rotation, elbow extension, forearm pronation, wrist extension with ulnar deviation, and finger extension (Fig. 78B). The therapist then moves MCs from the extensor surface of the hand, around the ulnar side of the hands into the palm to stretch and facilitate the withdrawal, or reverse thrust (Figs. 78C, 78D).

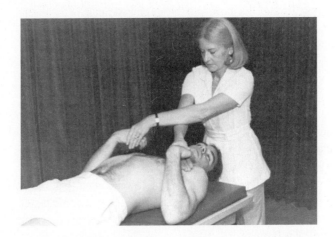

78A BS D1 thrust—lengthened range.

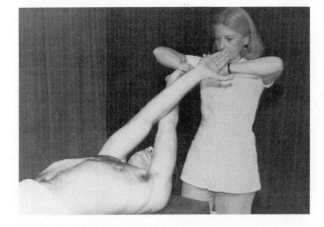

78B BS D1 thrust—shortened range.

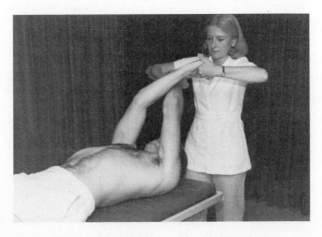

78C B2 D1 withdrawal—lengthened range.

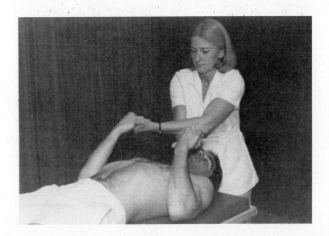

78D BS D1 withdrawal—shortened range.

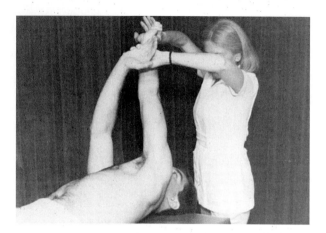

78E BS D1 thrust—TE thrust LUE.

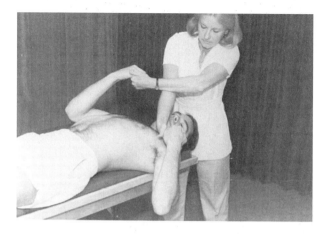

78F BS D1 withdrawal—TE withdrawal LUE.

To resist the pattern the arms are positioned in the lengthened range of the thrust as described, with the therapist's MCs on the extensor surface of the hand. Because the upper arm is on the plinth, stretch is applied primarily to the wrist and elbow components followed by resistance to all the components of the thrust. As the UEs move into the shortened range of the thrust the therapist steps back on the leg positioned posteriorly. The therapist's arms are raised and elbows flexed so the forearm of the therapist becomes an extension of the patient's arm. In the shortened range of the thrust, the hold is facilitated by an approximation force directed into the arm. For the reversal movement the MCs slide into the palms of the patient's hands and stretch, traction, and resistance are applied (Fig. 78C). As the patient moves into the shortened range of the withdrawal pattern, the therapist shifts weight onto the forward foot and the therapist's arms and elbows are extended and crossed (Fig. 78D). TE can be performed by locking in one arm in either the thrust or withdrawal pattern and pivoting the other. Movements that can be emphasized during the bilateral thrust are scapula protraction and shoulder flexion with adduction (Fig. 78E); during withdrawal, scapula retraction and shoulder extension can be reinforced (Fig. 78F).

The bilateral pattern can be performed reciprocally if the patient either reinforces better with this combination or if the patient's pattern of strength and weakness indicates that overflow would be better attained with a reciprocal pattern.

Thrust and withdrawal combine important proximal and distal movements.

Purpose/Treatment Goals

The purposes are to promote the combination of movements that occur in the thrust and withdrawal patterns and to specifically strengthen the serratus anterior, lower trapezius, anterior deltoid, and triceps (thrust) and middle trapezius, rhomboids, posterior deltoid, and wrist and finger flexors (withdrawal).

The combination of movements that occur in the thrust recombine the synergistic patterns and thus are appropriate for patients with dominant UE synergistic movements. To assist the hemiplegic patient in this pattern, the D1 thrust can be performed as a modified trunk pattern with the stronger arm holding onto the wrist of the weaker limb. Wrist and finger extension are promoted with the shoulder above 90 degrees of flexion (Souque's phenomenon). The thrusting movement also can be performed unilaterally in sidelying for patients who cannot overcome the effects of gravity (Fig. 78G).

For many athletes and other patients with orthopedic shoulder dysfunction improved control of scapula protraction and retraction are important. During the D1 thrust the serratus anterior and lower trapezius can be strengthened. Holding in the shortened range of the withdrawal

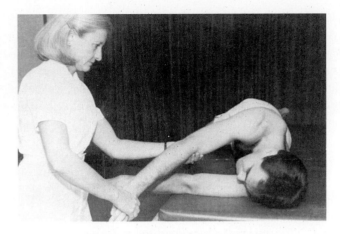

78G Unilateral thrust—shortened range.

motion enhances the rhomboids and middle trapezius. All of these scapular muscles are needed to decrease the tendency toward excessive winging or abduction of the scapula and to enhance proximal stability.

The withdrawal motion is similar to the movement of the UE in pivot prone. In this supine position the withdrawal movement is assisted by gravity, making the performance of this "modified pivot prone" procedure less difficult for many patients than the prone position.

Problems with Application

When resisting the thrusting pattern the therapist may not move with the patient's movement. The amount of scapula and shoulder motion may then be limited to approximately 90 degrees of flexion and range into shoulder adduction overemphasized.

The therapist may have difficulty controlling the thrust if full forearm pronation is allowed. As with most patterns, complete range of the rotational component should not occur.

Activity: Supine; BS D1F
Technique: Slow reversal hold (SRH); MC wrists

79

Description

In this supine position the BS D1 pattern is difficult for the therapist to control. With MCs on the wrists, full range into extension cannot be reached. In addition, the therapist loses control during the flexion motion as the patient's arms cross into adduction. Because the proximal components of this pattern are the same as the thrusting pattern, the thrust, which is performed with ease, is usually preferred.

Unilateral Upper Extremity

During these unilateral upper extremity procedures, the therapist must be careful with the placement of MCs, especially the distal contact. Because the hand is very sensitive to touch, proper contact is necessary to facilitate appropriate movement into finger flexion or extension.

The MCs are altered in a different manner with the UE patterns than with the LE. With the LE patterns, each contact remains in a distal or proximal position during the reversal movements. In the UE patterns, however, the proximal and distal contacts are usually interchanged as the reversal occurs. There are a few exceptions to this general rule, which will be mentioned as those patterns are discussed. As with all patterns it is important to guide the patient through the movement prior to adding any resistance. For all the following D2 patterns the *right* UE will be used as the example.

80

Activity: Supine; D2F elbow straight

Technique: Slow reversal hold (SRH); MC arm and hand

Impairments: Difficulty reversing movement; weakness in muscles of the flexor or extensor patterns; inappropriate timing of individual segments.

Individual muscle control can be achieved with unilateral patterns.

Description

The patient is positioned near the edge of the plinth with the therapist at the side. The limb is positioned in the lengthened range of D2F with the patient's thumb on the opposite hip. The therapist's left hand is placed on the extensor surface of the patient's wrist. This distal contact is positioned in a "lumbrical grip" with the thumb on the patient's fifth metacarpal and the fingers on the first metacarpal to ensure that no contact occurs in the palm of the hand. The right hand is positioned proximally on the upper arm. The forearm of the therapist's proximal contact is supinated and resistance is initially provided with the web space of that hand (Fig. 80A). The stretch applied with the proximal hand is primarily a traction and rotational force; the distal contact applies stretch to all the distal components. After the quick stretch, resistance is applied throughout the range of D2F. As the patient's UE moves into D2F, the therapist's forearm (proximal MC) remains supinated so the entire hand can resist the movement beyond 90 degrees of shoulder flexion. In the shortened range, holding is facilitated with either an approximation or traction force (Fig. 80B).

To reverse into D2E, the proximal contact moves into the patient's hand to resist wrist and finger flexion. This distal contact stretches the pattern with a traction rotational force (Fig. 80C). Once movement begins, the previously distal contact becomes the new proximal contact mov-

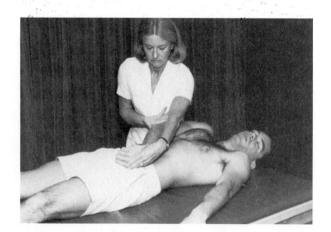

80A D2F—lengthened range.

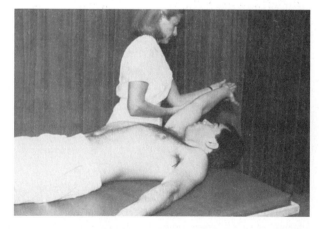

80B D2F—shortened range.

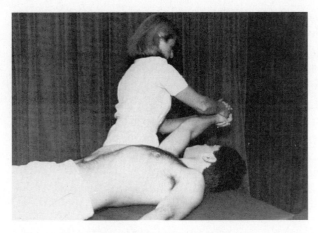

80C D2E—lengthened range.

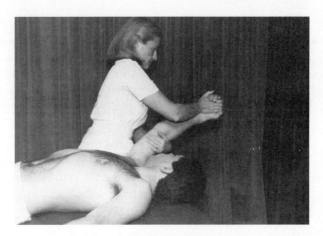

80D D2E—lengthened to mid range.

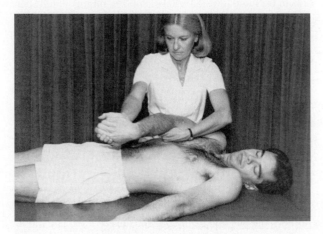

80E D2E—shortened range.

ing down toward the elbow approaching the arm from the medial side (Fig. 80D). In the shortened range of D2E the hold is facilitated with an approximation force (Fig. 80E). To reverse into D2F the proximal hand again becomes the distal contact on the extensor surface of the wrist. Stretch and resistance are applied and the new proximal contact is repositioned in supination on the upper arm. During these reversals the therapist's body rotates with the patient's UE movement to stay in the diagonal direction of the pattern. Verbal commands may be "open and turn your hand up and out to the side" (D2F), "hold it, now squeeze my hand and bring your arm down and across your body to your opposite hip" (D2E).

Purpose/Treatment Goals

The purposes are to facilitate the skill stage of control in the UE; to enhance the distal to proximal timing of movement; to promote a reversal of antagonists, and to strengthen the movements.

Control of the combination of movements that occurs in the unilateral D2F pattern is the goal for many patients. Shoulder flexion, abduction, and external rotation are the movements commonly limited (capsular pattern), therefore full range and smooth coordinated movement throughout range is desired.

For patients with neurological deficits this pattern recombines the synergistic movements: shoulder flexion and abduction with elbow extended. This is the most difficult combination of movements for many hemiplegic patients to perform. Normal control over this pattern, especially with the elbow and wrist maintained in extension, should not be expected until late in the rehabilitation process.

In this pattern the rotator cuff must control both the movement and the stability of the humerus within the glenoid fossa. In addition, for full shoulder flexion to occur, upward rotation of the scapula is required. Thus, for skilled unilateral movement, proximal dynamic stability is required in the scapula and the shoulder. To further challenge the patient, this pattern can be performed sitting where support is decreased and the effects of gravity are altered.

Problems with Application

Therapists may attempt to reposition the proximal contact too quickly, thereby losing the smooth reversal of antagonists. The therapist's motions should be smooth and rhythmical. Because the goal of this unilateral pattern is to promote the skill level of control, timing and proper sequencing of movement is emphasized. Unless strengthening of all or particular components of the pattern is the goal, resistance is minimal.

81

Activity: Supine; D2F, elbow flexing
Technique: Slow reversal hold (SRH); MC arm and hand
Impairments: Scapular and shoulder weakness.

Flexing the elbow shortens the lever arm and lessens the challenge to proximal muscles.

Description

In this activity the elbow flexes with shoulder flexion and extends with shoulder extension. The patient's position and the MCs begin in the same position as the previous procedure. The therapist's position, however, is more in the diagonal direction of the pattern, closer to the head of the plinth.

The pattern is stretched in the lengthened range of D2F. The stretch emphasizes the elbow flexors (Fig. 81A). The patient's movement into D2F with elbow flexion is resisted and the hand guided to the top of the head (Fig. 81B). To maintain resistance to the elbow flexion, the thera-

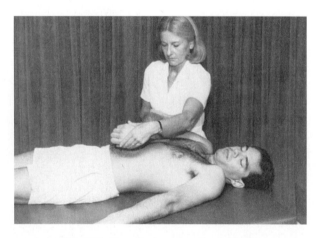

81A D2F, elbow flexing—lengthened range.

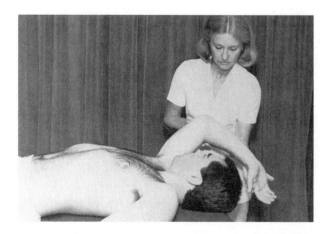

81B D2F, elbow flexing—shortened range.

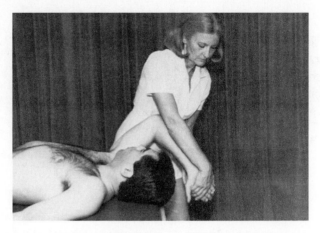

81C D2E, elbow extending—lengthened range.

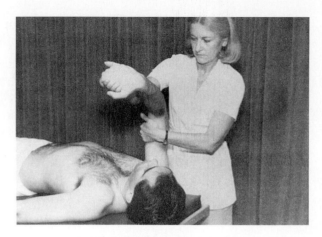

81D D2E, elbow extending—mid range.

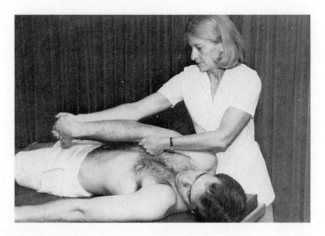

81E D2E, elbow extending—shortened range.

pist's fourth and fifth fingers are curled under the patient's wrist. The rest of the therapist's distal contact resists the wrist and finger extension by remaining on the extensor surface of the patient's hand. To reverse into D2E, the proximal contact moves into the patient's hand and the therapist's hand and forearm contact the patient's forearm. The distal contact stretches the pattern (Fig. 81C). As with stretch in other procedures, care must be taken not to stress the anterior shoulder. As the reverse D2E with elbow extending motion begins, the proximal contact is positioned near the patient's elbow (Fig. 81D). The proximal contact primarily resists the proximal components; the distal contact resists the forearm and distal components. In the shortened range of D2E, resistance to elbow extension is emphasized with an approximation force (Fig. 81E). Verbal commands may be "open your hand, bend your elbow, and bring your hand to the top of your head." "Now squeeze my hand and straighten your arm down to your opposite hip."

Purpose/Treatment Goals

The purposes are to combine the muscular activity of the middle deltoid and biceps in D2F and the sternal pectoralis major and triceps in D2E and to enhance activity of the supraspinatus and infraspinatus with a shortened lever arm. This pattern should be avoided with patients dominated by synergistic movements.

Problems with Application

The therapist may not resist elbow flexion adequately or throughout the full range. After 90 degrees of shoulder motion, if the therapist does not have the proper contact on the distal forearm to resist elbow flexion, a tendency exists to resist elbow extension instead of flexion.

The stretch into D2E is difficult for the therapist to control. Stretch may be given incorrectly to the elbow flexors or may overemphasize shoulder rotational movement. The correct stretch, which should not be forceful, is to both the sternal pectoralis major and the triceps.

82

Activity: Supine; D2F elbow extending
Technique: Slow reversal hold (SRH); MC arm and hand
Impairments: Scapular, shoulder and triceps weakness.

Description

In this pattern the elbow extends with shoulder flexion and flexes with shoulder extension. To begin the movement the patient is positioned with the arm in D2E and the elbow flexed so that the flexed hand is on the opposite shoulder. The therapist's left hand is on the extensor surface of the patient's right wrist and the proximal right contact is on the upper arm (Fig. 82A). A stretch is applied in the direction of further extension of the shoulder and flexion of the elbow and the wrist. The patient then moves into D2F extending the elbow throughout the range. This movement is resisted into the shortened range of the pattern where the elbow extension component is emphasized with resistance and approximation (Fig. 82B). To reverse to the antagonistic D2E pattern, *the distal contact remains distal and the proximal contact remains proximal.* The distal contact moves from the extensor surface of the wrist into the hand by pivoting around the fifth metacarpal or ulnar side of the hand. Stretch to D2E, primarily a traction rotational force is performed. The proximal MC is repositioned below the patient's elbow onto the volar surface and the reverse motion of shoulder extension with elbow flexion is resisted (Fig. 82C). Following the hold to this pattern, the distal contact again moves onto the extensor surface of the hand to stretch and resist the reversal motion, then the proximal MC moves to the upper arm. Verbal commands are "open your hand and straighten your elbow up over your head" (D2F). "Now squeeze my hand, bend your elbow and bring your hand toward your other shoulder" (D2E).

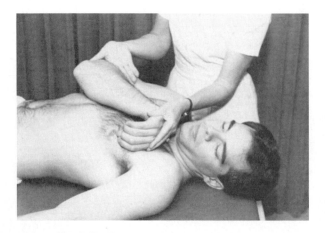

82A D2F, elbow extending—lengthened range.

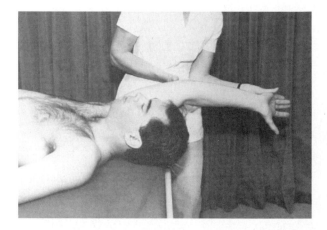

82B D2F, elbow extending—shortened range.

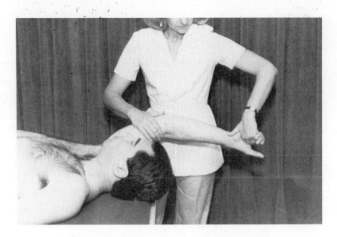

82C D2E, elbow flexing—lengthened range.

Purpose/Treatment Goals

The purpose is to combine the muscular activity of the middle deltoid with triceps and the sternal portion of the pectoralis major with the biceps.

The movement of shoulder flexion with elbow extension recombines the synergistic patterns and this is appropriate in the late stages of rehabilitation of hemiplegic patients. For patients with quadriplegia, this combination may be best to strengthen the triceps.

Problems with Application

During the extensor pattern, the patient may tend to bring the arm down to the side rather than to adduct the arm across the body. Verbal commands coupled with proper stretch, resistance, and placement of MCs must be used to promote the correct movement. This may be most evident in SCI patients who have decreased strength in the shoulder adductors. If this procedure is designed to enhance the activity of those specific muscles, then the adduction component of the pattern must be emphasized.

Activity: Supine; D1F, elbow straight

Technique: Slow reversal hold (SRH); MC arm and hand

Impairments: Difficulty reversing movements; weakness in muscles of the flexor or extensor patterns; inappropriate timing of segments.

83

Description

For all of the following D1 patterns, the *left* arm will be used as the example.

The patient is positioned near the edge of the plinth with the left arm in D1E. The therapist stands at the side facing the patient's hand. The therapist's right hand is in the patient's palm, thumb adjacent to thumb. The proximal contact is on the upper arm approaching it from the medial side to promote adduction of the shoulder (Fig. 83A). During the initiation of movement the therapist is cradling the patient's arm. A stretch to the flexion pattern is performed incorporating traction and rotation to the proximal components and a stretch to all the distal components. The arm is resisted into the shortened range of D1F along with the verbal command of

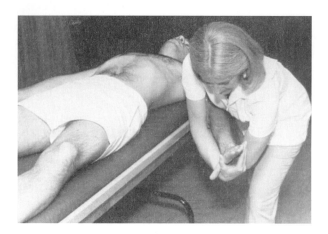

83A D1F—lengthened range.

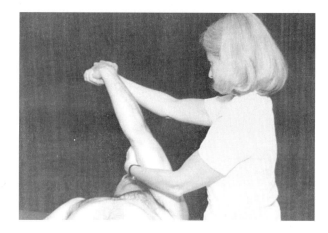

83B D1F—shortened range.

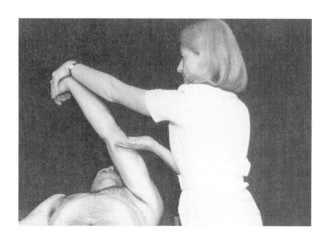

83C D2E—lengthened range.

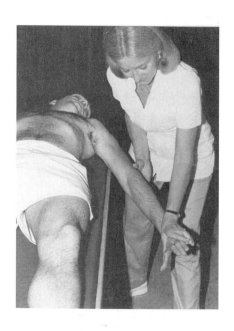

83D D2E—shortened range.

"squeeze my hand and move your arm up and across your face." The therapist pivots around to face the patient as the movement into D1F begins. An isometric contraction is performed in the shortened range of D1F (Fig. 83B). The proximal contact is then moved distally onto the extensor surface of the wrist and applies the stretch which incorporates traction and rotation. As the D1E pattern is initiated, what was the distal contact during the flexor movement is now shifted proximally and placed on the posterior surface of the upper arm from the lateral side (Fig. 83C). Verbal commands are "open your hand, turn and bring it down to your side." The hold in the shortened range of D1E combines resistance to all the components of the pattern as well as an approximation force (Fig. 83D). The proximal MC then returns to the hand and the distal contact moves proximally to once again stretch and resist the D1F pattern. Although this is a "straight arm" pattern, the elbow may have a tendency to flex slightly during the D1F movement.

Purpose/Treatment Goals

The purposes are to facilitate the skill stage of control; to enhance the proper distal to proximal timing of movement; to promote the reversal of antagonists; and to strengthen major muscle groups including the serratus anterior, anterior deltoid, biceps, and wrist and finger flexors (D1F), and the middle trapezius, rhomboids, posterior deltoid, triceps and wrist and finger extensors (D1E).

Problems with Application

If the patient pronates the forearm completely in the beginning of the D1E pattern, the therapist will lose control. Also, in the shortened range of D1E, too much rotation of the shoulder and forearm will prevent the therapist from maintaining the proper MC and giving resistance to all the components. As with all patterns, the individual components of the pattern do not always move through complete range.

Activity: Supine; D1F, elbow flexing
Technique: Slow reversal hold (SRH); MC arm and hand
Impairments: Scapular, shoulder, elbow, hand weakness; dominance of synergistic movements.

84

Description

The pattern is similar to the procedure just described and the therapist's position and placement of MCs are the same. In this activity, however, the elbow component is resisted throughout its range. When the stretch is applied to the flexion pattern, stretch to the elbow flexors is emphasized (Fig. 84A). The movement into elbow flexion is initiated at the beginning of the flexion pattern and is completed as the shortened range of the shoulder movement is reached (Fig. 84B). In this shortened range all components are resisted. The D1E pattern is then stretched and resisted. In this movement elbow extension occurs simultaneously along with the proximal and distal extension movements (Fig. 84C). Verbal commands are "squeeze my hand, bend your elbow and move your arm across your face (D1F)." "Now open your hand, straighten your elbow, and bring your arm down toward your side" (D1E).

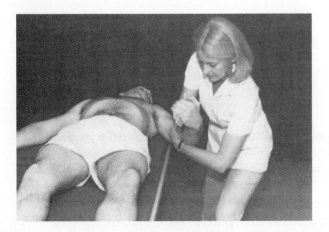

84A D1F, elbow flexing—lengthened range.

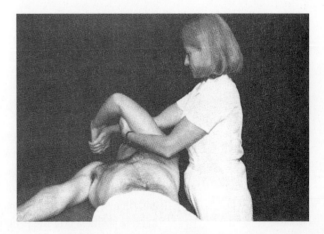

84B D1F, elbow flexing—shortened range.

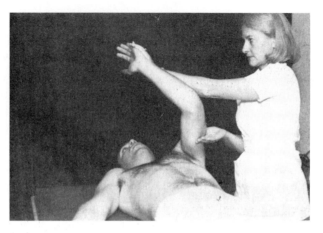

84C D1E, elbow extending—lengthened range.

Purpose/Treatment Goals

The purpose is to combine shoulder flexion and adduction with elbow flexion and shoulder extension and abduction with elbow extension to strengthen all of the muscles in the pattern. Increased emphasis is placed on the biceps and triceps contraction throughout the range of movement.

Problems with Application

The therapist may have difficulty controlling the correct sequencing of the pattern. The tendency of the patient is to flex the shoulder, then to flex the elbow, and in D1E to extend the elbow, then to extend the shoulder. The proximal and intermediate joints should move simultaneously, not sequentially. In addition, the therapist must be sure that the shoulder flexes and adducts appropriately across the body. The patient commonly flexes the elbow toward the face and leaves the shoulder in the midrange position.

In the lengthened range of D1E the therapist may have difficulty stretching the extensor pattern. Because the triceps are already lengthened at both joints, additional external stretch at the elbow may not be needed.

85

Activity: Supine; D1F, elbow extending
Technique: Slow reversal hold (SRH); MC arm and hand
Impairments: Scapular, shoulder, elbow and particularly wrist extensor weakness.

Description

In this pattern the elbow extends with shoulder flexion and flexes with shoulder extension. The patient is positioned at the size of the plinth and the therapist stands in the diagonal of the pattern at the side of the plinth facing the head of the patient. To begin the pattern the upper arm is hyperextended off the edge of the plinth, the elbow flexed with the forearm pronated and wrist and fingers extended. The back of the patient's hand is near the shoulder. The therapist's left hand is positioned in the patient's left palm and the right MC is positioned just above the elbow on the anterior surface of the arm (Fig. 85A). A stretch is applied to all components of the pat-

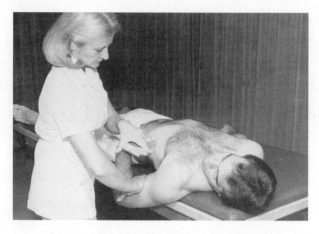

85A D1F, elbow extending—lengthened range.

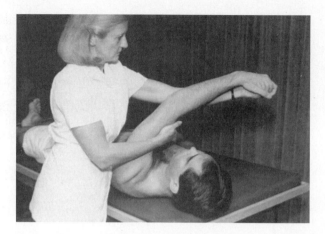

85B D1F, elbow extending—shortened range.

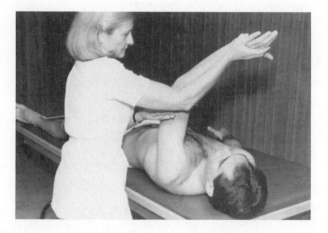

85C D1E, elbow flexing—lengthened range.

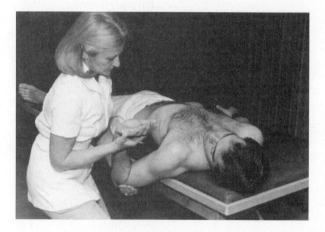

85D D1E, elbow flexing—shortened range.

tern. The patient flexes the wrist and the fingers, extends the elbow, and flexes the shoulder across the face. The distal contact emphasizes resistance to the elbow extension component and approximates through the limb as the isometric resistance is applied by both contacts in the shortened range (Fig. 85B). To reverse the pattern, the proximal contact moves distally and is positioned on the extensor surface of the wrist; the distal contact moves proximally to the posterior surface of the upper arm (Fig. 85C). The stretch is a traction force followed by resistance into the shortened range of D1E with the elbow flexing (Fig. 85D).

Purpose/Treatment Goals

The purposes are to combine shoulder flexion with elbow extension (anterior deltoid with triceps) and wrist flexion and shoulder extension with elbow flexion (posterior deltoid with biceps) and wrist extension; to strengthen all of the muscles in the pattern. Wrist extensors, in particular, appear to be easily facilitated with this combination of movements.

    Although in most cases the thrust pattern previously described is easier for the therapist to control and for the patient to perform, there are certain patients for whom this activity is more appropriate, e.g., SCI patients with quadriplegia.

    In this pattern, similar to that of withdrawal, shoulder hyperextension and internal rotation

Wrist extension is easily facilitated when combined with shoulder extension and elbow flexion.

can be emphasized. For a quadriplegic this motion is important to strengthen the muscles that will help the patient assume supine on elbows.

Problems with Application

During the flexion pattern, resistance to flexion of the wrist and hand in conjunction with elbow extension may be difficult. In this direction, however, the elbow rather than the distal component is the movement usually emphasized.

86

Activity: Supine; unilateral D1 thrust, shortened or lengthened range of emphasis

Technique: Slow reversal hold (SRH) with timing for emphasis (TE); MC arm and hand

Impairments: Weakness in shortened or lengthened range of muscles in either the thrust or withdrawal pattern.

Description

The therapist can be positioned at either end of the pattern; at the head of the plinth to best resist the shortened range of the thrust and the lengthened range of the withdrawal pattern or at the side of the plinth to best resist the shortened range of the withdrawal and the lengthened range of the thrust pattern.

With the therapist standing at the head of the plinth, the patient's left arm is positioned in the lengthened range of the thrust, in shoulder extension, elbow flexion, with the fisted hand anterior to the shoulder. The therapist's right contact is on the extensor surface of the patient's left hand and the left contact is proximal to the patient's elbow on the anterior surface of the arm (Fig. 86A). Stretch is applied to all the components of the pattern followed by resistance to the thrusting movement into the shortened range. During this movement the therapist rocks back onto the posterior foot and moves with the patient's movement to allow the shoulder to move into flexion across the patient's face. The hold in the shortened range is primarily an approximation force attempting to "collapse" the limb (Fig. 86B). To reverse the pattern, *the distal contact stays distal* but moves around the ulnar border of the hand into the palm to resist wrist and finger flexion. The stretch to the withdrawal motion is largely a traction force. As the withdrawal pattern is initiated, the proximal hand moves to the posterior surface of the upper arm to resist the proximal component (Figs. 86C, 86D). As with the bilateral thrust, the therapist must move with the patient's movement, otherwise the shoulder adduction component during the thrust will be overemphasized and range into shoulder flexion limited.

Proper positioning of the therapist is necessary to provide adequate resistance in the weakened part of the range.

If imbalances of muscle strength exist within the thrust pattern, the technique of TE can be used. For example, to emphasize the **serratus anterior** or the motion of scapular protraction and upward rotation, the thrust pattern is resisted into the shortened range of shoulder flexion. The stronger components are locked in by adding approximation to the isometric contraction. Scapula protraction is then emphasized as the scapula is pivoted off the plinth. Verbal commands are "lift your arm up (resisting the thrust), "hold it" (locking in the stronger components) and "reach up toward the ceiling" (pivoting or adding repeated contractions to scapula protraction).

To emphasize the **anterior deltoid** and the shoulder movement of flexion, adduction, and external rotation, the arm is flexed to the point of weakness where the stronger triceps and distal components are locked in. The shoulder motions are then pivoted.

The **triceps** can also be strengthened by locking in the proximal and distal components and pivoting the intermediate elbow joint (Fig. 86E).

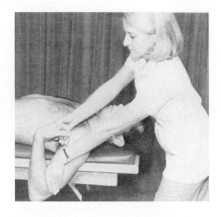

86A D1 thrust—lengthened range.

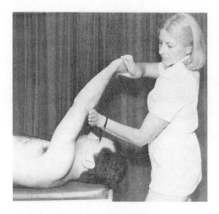

86B D1 thrust—shortened range.

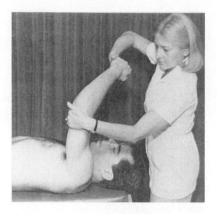

86C D1 withdrawal—lengthened range.

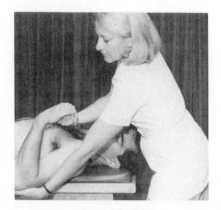

86D D1 withdrawal—shortened range.

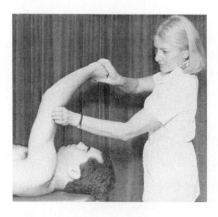

86E D1 thrust—TE elbow extension.

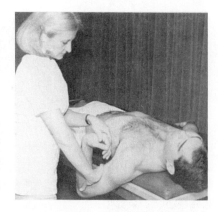

86F D1 thrust—lengthened range.

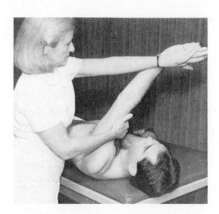

86G D1 thrust—shortened range.

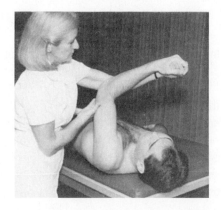

86H D1 withdrawal—lengthened range

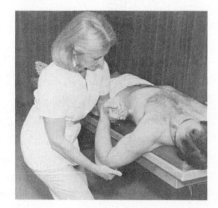

86I D1 withdrawal—shortened range.

As stated, the position of the therapist is at the side of the plinth when the emphasis of the procedure is either the shortened range of the withdrawal pattern or the lengthened range of the thrust. The therapist's left distal contact is positioned distally on the extensor surface of the patient's hand, and the proximal contact on the anterior surface of the patient's arm proximal to the elbow (Fig. 86F). The entire pattern is stretched and resisted into the shortened range of the thrust (Fig. 86G). To reverse into the withdrawal pattern, the distal contact remains distal and moves into the palmar surface of the hand (Figs. 86H, 86I). An alternate and equally effective

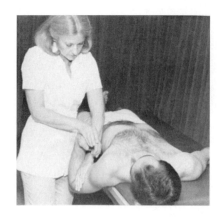

86J D1 thrust—lengthened range.

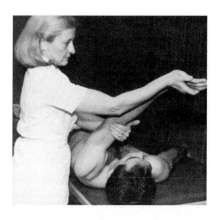

86K D1 thrust—shortened range.

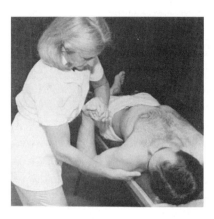

86L D1 withdrawal—TE scapular retraction.

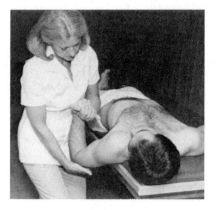

86M D1 withdrawal—TE shoulder hyperextension.

method is to reverse proximal and distal contacts during the thrust movement (Figs. 86J, 86K).

Strengthening of the rhomboids and the posterior deltoid in the shortened range can be accomplished in the withdrawal pattern with the therapist in this position. To facilitate the **rhomboids** the therapist's proximal hand is moved onto the posterior surface of the scapula to provide resistance to scapula retraction. The distal contact resists and locks in the shoulder, elbow, and hand components as the proximal contact pivots the scapular retraction (Fig. 86L).

To emphasize the **posterior deltoid,** the elbow, wrist, and finger flexors are locked in by the distal contact. The proximal hand positioned on the posterior surface of the upper arm resists the movement into shoulder hyperextension (Fig. 86M).

Purpose/Treatment Goals

The purpose is to strengthen specific muscles in either lengthened or shortened ranges within either the thrust or the withdrawal pattern.

The distal components also can be emphasized during these patterns. Wrist extension in the thrust pattern can be pivoted above 90 degrees of shoulder flexion. Wrist flexion activity enhanced by overflow from the elbow flexors can be pivoted during withdrawal.

The range into hyperextension is important for many patients to improve their ability to reach behind their back.

Problems with Application

The therapist needs to move with the pattern to control the movement of the patient. If the therapist remains stationary the diagonal direction and complete range of the pattern may be compromised.

In the following procedures the techniques of TE or RC will be emphasized to strengthen specific muscles or to reinforce the proximal, intermediate, or distal components of the pattern. Techniques to increase contractile tissue extensibility, i.e., HR or CR, will be incorporated into the procedures. The skill level of function will be promoted with the technique of NT. Review the previous procedures for the therapist's position and placement of manual contacts.

Activity: Supine; D1F, elbow flexing

Technique: Slow reversal hold (SRH) with timing for emphasis (TE) on shoulder, elbow; MC arm and hand

Impairments: Weakness of shoulder flexors, adductors, or elbow flexors.

87

Description

In the D1F pattern the anterior deltoid, pectoralis major, and biceps can be specifically emphasized. To enhance anterior deltoid and the clavicular portion of the **pectoralis major** the stronger biceps and wrist and finger flexors are "locked in" at approximately 90 degrees and the weaker shoulder muscles are pivoted (Fig. 87A). To strengthen the **biceps,** the proximal and distal components are "locked in" at midrange and the biceps are pivoted.

Purpose/Treatment Goals

The purpose is to strengthen the anterior deltoid and pectoralis major or the biceps by promoting overflow from the stronger components within the pattern.

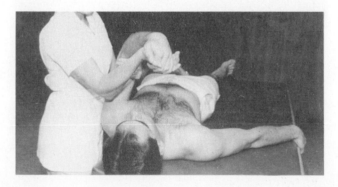

87A D1F, elbow flexing—TE shoulder.

88

Activity: Supine; D2E, elbow flexing

Technique: Slow reversal (SR) with timing for emphasis (TE) on the shoulder, elbow; MC arm and hand

Impairments: Weakness of shoulder extensors, adductors, elbow flexors.

Description

In this procedure the stronger biceps can be used to promote overflow to the weaker sternal portion of the **pectoralis major** (Fig. 88A). The pattern is initiated with stretch and resistance from the lengthened range of D2E. The biceps and distal components are locked in their midranges. The pectoralis major is then pivoted emphasizing the movement of the arm adducting across the body and the elbow moving toward the umbilicus. If the sternal pectoralis is stronger than the biceps, then the pectoralis would be locked in near its shortened range and the biceps pivoted.

Purpose/Treatment Goals

The purpose is to strengthen the sternal portion of the pectoralis major by promoting overflow from the elbow, wrist, and fingers or to strengthen the biceps when the sternal portion of the pectoralis is the strongest muscle at the shoulder.

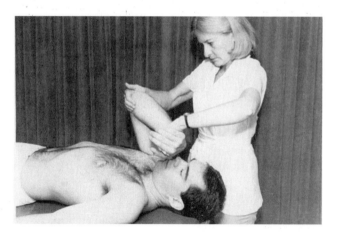

88A D2E, elbow flexing—TE shoulder.

Activity: Supine; D2F, elbow extending

Technique: Slow reversal hold (SRH) with timing for emphasis (TE) on elbow extension; MC arm and hand

Impairments: Weakness of elbow extensors.

89

Description

In this activity the stronger middle deltoid and wrist extensors are "locked in" with the shoulder above 90 degrees and the **triceps** are pivoted (Fig. 89A). If the triceps are very weak, holding in the shortened range of elbow extension and resistance from the mid to shortened range can be emphasized before movement throughout the range. In this range, gravity may be less of a resistive factor and lengthened ranges can be avoided. When the triceps are stronger, resistance can be applied throughout the entire range of elbow extension.

Purpose/Treatment Goals

The purpose is to enhance the activity of the triceps by overflow from the stronger middle deltoid and the wrist and finger extensors.

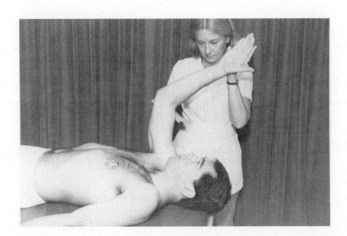

89A D2F, elbow extending—TE triceps.

90

Activity: Supine; D2F elbow straight
Technique: Slow reversal hold (SRH) with repeated contractions (RC); MC arm and hand
Impairments: Weakness of any muscle active in D2F.

Description

The technique of RC applied to a straight arm pattern promotes strengthening of all of the muscles in the pattern but particularly the proximal components. RC is applied by giving quick stretch and resistance throughout the range if weakness is equal throughout. If weakness is primarily in the shortened range of the pattern, an isometric contraction can be applied just prior to the point of weakness to facilitate alpha gamma coactivation. Following this hold, quick stretch and resistance are added to promote an increase in muscular activity into the shortened range.

Purpose/Treatment Goals

The purpose is to strengthen the trapezius, middle deltoid, supraspinatus, infraspinatus, and other muscles active in the D2F pattern.

91

Sidelying mini-mizes the effects of gravity on proximal muscles.

Activity: Sidelying, supine; scapular protraction with shoulder flexion
Technique: Hold relax active movement (HRAM); guided agonistic reversals (AR); MC scapula and arm
Impairments: Weakness or abnormal tone in scapular or shoulder muscles.

Description

This procedure develops initial proximal mobility in the UE. The progression is from sidelying to supine to increase the effects of gravity. The patient is first positioned in sidelying with the therapist's MCs on the lateral border of the scapula and on the arm. The patient's hand can be secured around the therapist's elbow. The modified technique of HRAM begins by protracting the scapula. In the shortened range a gentle holding contraction is facilitated. Following the relaxation of this contraction the scapula is slowly stretched into a slightly lengthened range of the protractors and active movement is guided back into the shortened range. As control of the protractors is gained, both the range and the strength of the contraction are increased. The shoulder flexors are facilitated in a similar manner. The limb is moved into 90 degrees of flexion where a holding contraction is facilitated. Relaxation is followed by stretch and active movement into flexion.

In supine, gravity resists these movements. The technique of AR can be performed with MCs assisting the limb movement. The procedure begins with the shoulder flexed to 90 degrees. Concentric scapula protraction is facilitated with one MC under the scapula and the other helping to support the weight of the limb. When the shortened range is reached, the eccentric contraction is assisted through increments of range. By progressing one joint more distally, control of the shoulder flexion follows with eccentric–concentric contractions. Gentle lowering of the limb from 90 degrees of flexion to the side is allowed. If the patient begins to lose control, the limb is assisted concentrically back to the starting 90-degree position.

Purpose/Treatment Goals

The purpose is to facilitate scapular protraction and shoulder flexion.

These procedures are appropriate with patients demonstrating synergistic patterns of movement or extreme weakness or pain secondary to trauma or surgery. The level of patient effort must be monitored to ensure normal muscular responses. The amount of effort is gradually increased by first eliminating gravity then moving the patient into a gravity resisted position.

Problems with Application

Excessive effort by the patient may cause abnormal reactions. The trunk and the limbs are repositioned and moved cautiously to avoid these responses.

Activity: Sitting; unilateral UE movements

Technique: Hold after positioning (placing); agonistic reversals (AR); MC arm and forearm

Impairments: Inability to control arm movements through a 90-degree arc in upright postures.

92

Descriptions

Control of unilateral UE movements can be promoted with these procedures. The limb is guided into shoulder flexion with the elbow maintained in extension. At 90 degrees of flexion the assistance is withdrawn and the patient holds the limb in that position. Following this isometric contraction in shortened ranges, eccentric–concentric contractions are performed. If any loss of control is detected as the patient slowly lowers the arm, the arm is assisted back to the starting 90-degree position. To increase the difficulty of the procedure the shoulder can be positioned in more abduction and the forearm supinated while maintaining the elbow in an extended position.

Purpose/Treatment Goals

The purpose is to improve isometric holding and concentric–eccentric control against gravitational resistance.

For patients demonstrating synergistic patterns the goal is to promote individualized movement or to recombine synergistic combinations. These movements may be promoted first in sidelying and supine as described in the previous procedure, then progressed to the sitting posture where the challenge to limb movement is further increased.

Problems with Application

The therapist may attempt this activity before control in less stressful postures has been developed. Too little assistance to the arm may increase the amount of patient effort to the extent that abnormal reactions or compensatory movements occur. The patient must have sufficient trunk balance in the sitting posture before extremity control can be developed.

93

Activity: Supine; D2F, elbow straight
Technique: Hold relax (HR), contract relax (CR); MC arm and hand
Impairments: Decreased shoulder mobility (ROM) in the D2 direction.

Mobility techniques promote ROM in conjunction with strengthening weakened agonists.

Description

The techniques of HR and CR can be used to increase the extensibility of the contractile tissues. The procedures described can lengthen the muscles that are the prime movers in the D2E pattern thus increasing movement into D2F.

HR can be performed with the isometric contraction applied either to the agonist (D2F pattern) or the antagonist (D2E pattern). The choice of HR to the agonist is preferred because the flexor pattern can be facilitated while the extensor pattern is simultaneously inhibited through reciprocal inhibition.

The D2F pattern is resisted to the point of limitation where an isometric contraction of all the muscles in this pattern is performed. The contraction is slowly increased until a moderate level of tension is achieved; relaxation follows, with the therapist supporting the limb. The therapist then facilitates active motion into the new range with resistance to tolerance. The technique is repeated until no additional range is gained. The alternative of applying HR to the antagonistic muscles of the D2E pattern also may result in inhibition. However, the secondary goal of activating the agonist is not simultaneously accomplished with this method.

Unlike HR, CR is always performed to the antagonistic or range-limiting pattern in the following manner: the D2F pattern is resisted to the point of limitation, MCs are changed and resistance is applied to the muscles of the D2E pattern. Isometric resistance to the extensor and adductor components is combined with isotonic resistance to the rotational component. The verbal commands are brisk and energetic, "turn your arm and pull down toward your opposite hip." The contraction builds quickly to a maximum level. When maximum tension is achieved or when the rotational component is completed, relaxation is allowed. MCs are reversed again and movement into the newly gained range of D2F is then minimally resisted.

Purpose/Treatment Goals

The purposes are to promote the mobility stage of control; to gain ROM into D2F by increasing the extensibility of the range-limiting muscles; and to strengthen the muscles in the D2F pattern.

Range into D2F or the capsular pattern of shoulder flexion, abduction, and external rotation commonly is limited. Decreased extensibility may be found in both the contractile and noncontractile tissues. To affect the noncontractile tissues, joint mobilization and thermal modalities are most effective; for the contractile tissues, the techniques of HR or CR are appropriate.

Problems with Application

The therapist may not allow complete relaxation to occur before asking for active movement of the agonistic pattern. If the patient complains of pain, additional time must be allowed for relaxation.

During the technique of HR the therapist may use improper verbal commands that will elicit isotonic contractions. Verbal commands such as "hold" or "don't let me move you," which evoke an isometric contraction should accompany this technique.

Activity: Supine; scapular patterns either bilateral or unilateral

Technique: Hold relax (HR), rhythmic stabilization (RS), slow reversal hold (SRH); MC scapula

Impairments: Decreased scapular mobility and stability.

94

Description

The therapist stands at the head of the plinth facing the patient. HR can be performed to increase range of scapular motions and to decrease abnormal tension in the scapular muscles. To promote relaxation of the upper trapezius, HR can be applied to the agonistic scapular depressors as well as directly to the antagonistic scapular elevators. The isometric contraction is slowly increased followed by relaxation and then movement into scapular depression. In conjunction with the procedure, slow deep breathing may be incorporated to further increase the relaxation response.

If the patient demonstrates tightness in the pectoralis minor and the scapula is depressed and anteriorly tilted, HR can be applied to improve scapular elevation and adduction. MCs are placed over the anterior shoulder and HR is applied directly to the tight muscle.

RS promotes isometric contractions of both scapulae and can be used to enhance relaxation or promote proximal stability. MCs are positioned to apply resistance in opposite directions. This procedure indirectly promotes isometric contractions of the shoulder musculature and is thus appropriate for patients with shoulder pain.

Once range and relaxation have been achieved, SRH can be applied to enhance a smooth reversal of antagonists. This technique can be applied to movement in a straight line or to the diagonal patterns of the scapula. In the D1F pattern, the scapular protracts (elevation, abduction, and upward rotation); the prime mover is the serratus anterior (Fig. 94A). In D1E the scapula retracts (depression, adduction, and downward rotation); the prime mover is the rhomboids (Fig. 94B). Verbal commands may be "bring your shoulder up toward your nose" (D1F), and "pinch your shoulder blades together" (D1E). The D2F pattern combines scapular elevation, adduction, and upward rotation; the trapezius is the prime mover (Fig. 94C).

D2E combines scapular depression, abduction, and downward rotation; the pectoralis minor is the prime mover (Fig. 94D). Verbal commands for scapular movement in D2 may be "bring your shoulders up toward your ears" (D2F), and "curl your shoulders down and forward" (D2E).

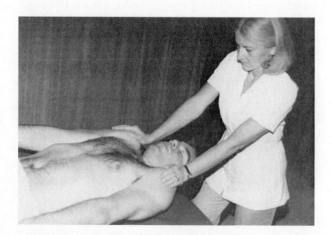

94A D1F—scapular elevation, abduction, upward rotation.

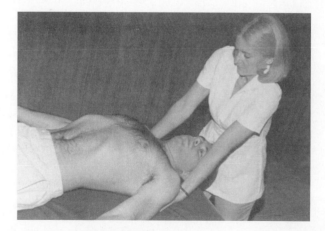

94B D1E—scapular depression, adduction, downward rotation.

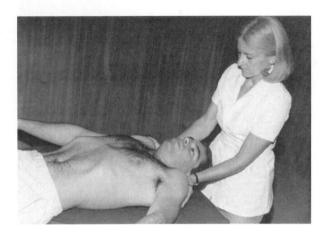

94C D2F—scapular elevation, adduction, upward rotation.

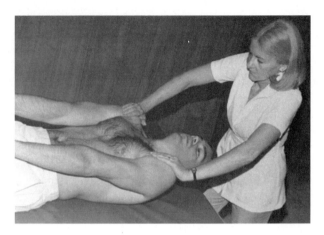

94D D2E—scapular depression, abduction, downward rotation.

Scapular patterns can be performed independently and in conjunction with diagonal shoulder movements.

Purpose/Treatment Goals

The purposes are to increase scapular ROM; to decrease tension of scapular muscles; to improve proximal stability; to facilitate a reversal of proximal muscles.

Many patients demonstrating tension in the upper trapezius also show tightness in the pectoralis minor. Extensibility of the anterior muscles should be assessed and treated.

Patients with pain in the upper extremity frequently protect the limb and hold the scapula elevated. In these cases the relaxation techniques applied proximally may decrease tension throughout the limb. With MCs on the scapula, massage can be easily incorporated into treatment.

Problems with Application

Therapists may have the patient contract too strongly or may not allow sufficient time for relaxation to occur. If pain is a symptom, allowing time for relaxation is especially important.

95

Both gravity and manual resistance are combined to strengthen proximal muscles in prone.

Activity: Prone; D1E, D2F

Technique: Slow reversal hold (SRH) with timing for emphasis (TE) to the scapula; MC arm and scapula

Impairments: Strength of shoulder and scapular muscles not less than 3/5.

Description

The patient is prone with the *right* arm over the side edge of the plinth. The two patterns that incorporated shoulder abduction, D2F and D1E, can be performed easily in prone. The focus of the procedure is primarily on the scapula and the shoulder. The proximal contact is positioned on the scapula, the distal contact is on the upper arm. The therapist is positioned in the diagonal direction of the pattern lateral to the patient's UE.

To resist D1E of the RUE the left contact is on the posterior upper arm and the right contact is on the scapula with the fingers on the scapula pointing caudally. The D1E pattern is stretched and resisted into the shortened range (Fig. 95A). The scapula retracts and the shoulder extends. To reverse into D1F, the distal contact remains distal but changes to the anterior

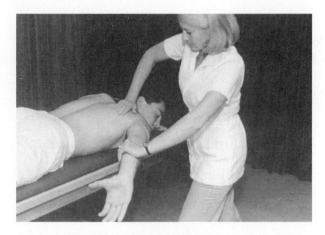

95A D1E—shortened range.

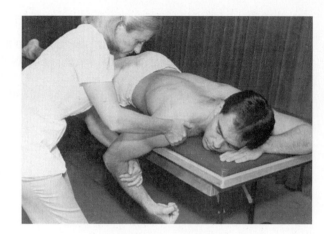

95B D1F—mid range.

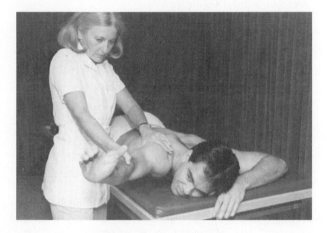

95C D2F—shortened range.

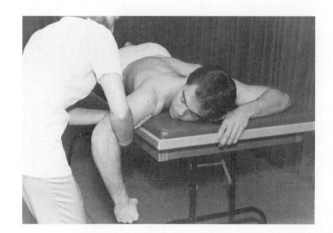

95D D2E—mid range.

arm to stretch and resist flexion and adduction of the shoulder. The proximal contact moves onto the anterior surface of the shoulder over the acromion process to resist scapular protraction (Fig. 95B).

To facilitate the rhomboids, TE is performed with emphasis on the scapula in D1E. The arm is locked in extension and the scapula pivoted into retraction. As the scapula moves into the shortened range, the arm must move an equal amount so as not to overstretch the isometrically contracting muscles of the shoulder. TE also can be applied to shoulder hyperextension to strengthen the posterior deltoid. Although more easily performed in other postures, TE can be applied to the flexion pattern to facilitate the serratus anterior or the anterior deltoid.

To resist D2F, the therapist's left contact is positioned on the scapula near the acromion process, the right contact is on the upper arm (Fig. 95C). The emphasis can be on either the shoulder or the scapular motion. To reverse the pattern, the distal contact again remains distal, moving under the upper arm, and the proximal contact moves into the axilla (Fig. 95D). Resistance can then be applied to the scapula and the shoulder in D2E. Adduction is limited by the supporting surface in both the D1F and D2E directions.

Purpose/Treatment Goals

The purpose is to strengthen the shoulder and scapular muscles in the prone position where the gravitational and tonal effects differ from other more frequently used postures such as supine or sitting.

These patterns are very useful for patients who must remain prone for an extended time.

Problems with Application

The therapist may be positioned incorrectly between the patient's arm and body during the D1E pattern, forcing the shoulder into excessive abduction. The proper position for the therapist in both patterns is lateral to the patient's arm.

Utilizing the patterns already described, the next procedures demonstrate how the distal components of the UE can be facilitated and strengthened. *Manual contacts must be always positioned above and below the joint of emphasis.* The patient's upper arm may be stabilized on the plinth so that the therapist can better control the distal segments.

96

Activity: Supine; D1F, elbow flexing

Technique: Timing for emphasis (TE) on wrist, MCP, PIP and DIP flexion, thumb adduction; MC as needed

Impairments: Weakness of radial wrist and finger flexors; weakness of thumb adduction.

Description

In the D1F pattern, radial wrist flexion is promoted by locking in the proximal components, primarily the biceps, and pivoting the wrist flexion motion. MCs are placed above and below the joint to be emphasized: on the forearm (proximal contact) and in the hand (distal contact) (Fig. 96A). To promote MCP flexion the proximal contact moves to the hand and the distal contact to the fingers. To ensure only MCP flexion the PIPs are maintained in extension by the therapist's thumb (Fig. 96B). To promote PIP flexion the distal hand is on the middle phalanx and the proximal hand on the proximal phalanx (Fig. 96C). Movement of the DIPs can be performed by mov-

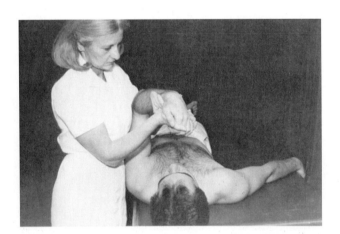
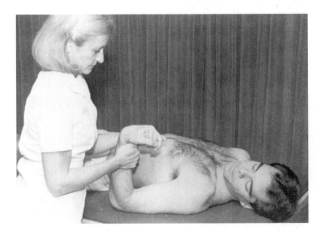

96A D1F, elbow flexion—TE wrist flexion.

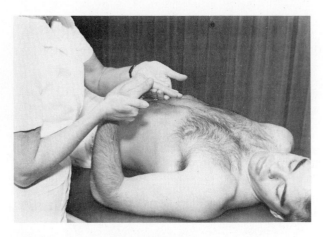

96B D1F, elbow flexion—TE MCP joints.

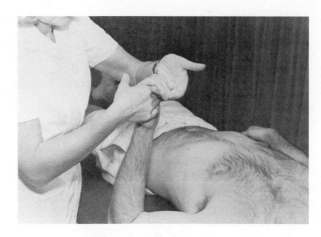

96C D1F, elbow flexion—TE PIP joints.

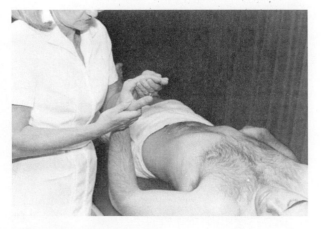

96D D1F, elbow flexion—TE thumb adduction.

ing the contacts to the middle and distal phalanx. Flexion of each finger can be performed separately or all four fingers can be moved simultaneously. The therapist can promote specific joint movement with the contacts just described or can resist the total finger flexion motion with the distal contact on the patient's fingertips. Thumb adduction also occurs in the D1F pattern. To enhance this motion the proximal contact is in the patient's hand and the distal contact on the patient's first metacarpal (Fig. 96D).

TE can be used to strengthen specific distal muscles.

Purpose/Treatment Goals

The purpose is to facilitate the specific movements of the hand that occur in the D1F pattern. Techniques applied to these movements will facilitate various aspects of control; TE will promote strengthening, HR can increase range of motion of the contractile tissues, and SR (SRH) will enhance the reversal movements of the flexors and extensors.

Problems with Application

When pivoting the carpal–metacarpal joint the therapist's MC should be on the first metacarpal so that forces are not transmitted through the MCP or the distal joint rather than the CMC joint.

97

Activity: Supine; D1E, elbow straight or flexing

Technique: Timing for emphasis (TE) on wrist and finger extension; MC as needed

Impairments: Weakness of ulnar wrist and finger extensors.

Description

In this activity, ulnar wrist extension, extension and abduction primarily of the fourth and fifth fingers, and abduction of the thumb can be promoted. The elbow can be "locked in" either in flexion (preferable) (Fig. 97A), or in extension (Fig. 97B), whichever best facilitates the distal musculature. As in the previous procedure the MCs are placed to promote control in one specific joint.

Purpose/Treatment Goals

The purpose is to facilitate the movements of the wrist, fingers, and thumb, that are activated in the D1E pattern.

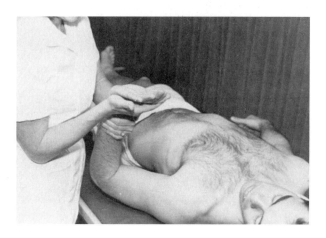

97A D1E—elbow flexion.

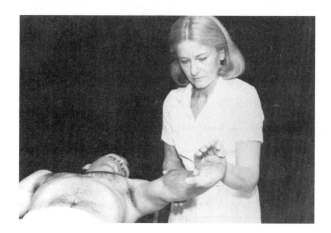

97B D1E—elbow straight.

98

Activity: Supine; D2E, elbow straight

Technique: Timing for emphasis (TE) on wrist and finger flexion, thumb opposition; MC as needed

Impairments: Weakness of ulnar wrist and finger flexors and thumb opposition.

Description

In the D2E pattern, movement of the ulnar wrist flexors and flexion of the first two fingers and thumb opposition can be promoted. The upper arm can be positioned on the plinth with the elbow flexed (Fig. 98A) or the shoulder can be locked in at approximately 90 degrees with the elbow straight. When emphasizing opposition, forearm pronation will help facilitate the rotation of the thumb. For thumb opposition, one MC is in the palm and the other is positioned proximally on the metacarpal to reduce the rotational torque at the first MCP (Fig. 98B).

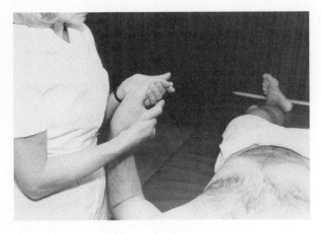

98A D2E—elbow flexed—TE forearm pronation.

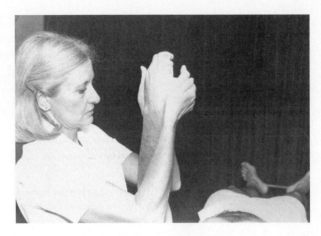

98B D2E—TE thumb opposition.

Purpose/Treatment Goals

The purpose is to facilitate the movements of the wrist, fingers, and thumb, that are active in the D2E pattern.

Activity: Supine; D2F, elbow straight or flexing

Technique: Timing for emphasis (TE) and normal timing (NT) on distal components; MC as needed

Impairments: Weakness of radial wrist and thumb extensors.

99

Description

In the D2F pattern, the radial wrist extension and the extension of the first two fingers and thumb can be facilitated. Abduction of the first and second finger also can be promoted. The first dorsal interossei can be facilitated in this pattern. As with the D2E pattern, the arm can be stabilized on the plinth or can be locked in at 90 degrees of the D2F pattern with the elbow straight.

The technique of NT is performed to combine wrist and finger extension in the initiation of the D2F pattern. To perform this procedure the therapist stands on the side opposite the limb to be facilitated. The entire pattern is stretched but the therapist limits the proximal movement until the distal movement is completed. First the wrist motion is promoted, then finger extension is added to the wrist motion.

Purpose/Treatment Goals

The purpose is to strengthen the movements that occur in the D2F pattern.

Once strength is achieved, NT of distal extension with the rest of the limb movement can be emphasized. Many patients can extend the wrist only when the arm is above 90 degrees of shoulder flexion. The goals for these patients would be to initiate the distal component in the lengthened range.

The interossei, the stabilizers of the fingers, can be facilitated in each of the four patterns described above. The interossei that abduct the fingers can be enhanced in the D1E pattern (third and fourth fingers) and the D2F pattern (first and second fingers). During hand rehabilitation these abduction motions of the fingers are combined with the finger extension that occurs in these patterns. The interossei that adduct the fingers are facilitated in the patterns where the fingers flex; in D2E the first and second fingers and in D1F the fourth and fifth fingers.

100

Activity: Supine; D1E, elbow straight

Technique: Rhythmic stabilization (RS); MC forearm, wrist, hand

Impairments: Poor stability in wrist; decreased mobility of distal musculature; pain or marked proximal weakness.

Description

In the supine position with the arm at the side in the D1E pattern, the technique of RS can be performed. MCs are positioned on the ulna and the radius (Fig. 100A). Isometric resistance is applied alternately to the forearm motions of supination and pronation. If increased ROM of forearm rotation is the goal, further movement into the desired range is allowed following the isometric contractions. MCs also can be positioned on the wrist or the hand to promote range or stability at those joints (Fig. 100B).

Purpose/Treatment Goals

The purpose is to promote stability in the radio-ulnar joint or more distally; to increase ROM; to indirectly facilitate proximal muscles, especially the rotator cuff.

Because of the gradual increase of isometric contractions, this procedure is particularly useful when pain is present.

The remaining procedures promote movement of the head and the neck and the facial and tongue muscles. Head and neck motions have already been incorporated into the upper trunk patterns of a chop and a lift. In the following procedures these motions are specifically promoted. The therapist must be careful during the extension patterns not to move into neck hypertension to avoid comprising circulation or increasing nerve impingement.

RS can be applied distally to relax painful proximal muscles.

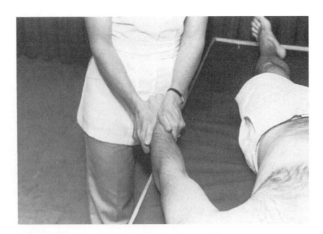

100A D1E —RS MC forearm.

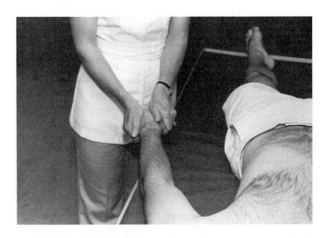

100B D1E—RS MC hand.

Head and Neck Patterns

101

Activity: Supine, sitting, or prone on elbows; head and neck patterns

Technique: Slow reversal hold (SRH), rhythmic stabilization (RS), hold relax (HR); MC head and chin

Impairments: Restricted mobility of cervical movements; pain or weakness in cervical muscles; decreased righting reactions; inadequate upper trunk or shoulder stability.

Description

Head and neck patterns can be performed in either supine, sitting, or prone on elbows (P on E) to facilitate diagonal head and neck flexion and extension with rotation or just rotation. Head motion performed primarily by the short neck flexors and extensors occurs in the superior region of the cervical spine; neck motion performed primarily by the longer flexors and extensors occurs lower in the cervical spine. Jaw opening is combined with neck flexion and jaw closing with neck extension.

In the supine position, the movement is performed with the head supported off the edge of the plinth so that extension can be accomplished. One MC is on the crown of the head. During the patient's movements this contact pivots on the head so that forearm supination occurs during extension and pronation during flexion. The other MC is on the inferior or superior surface of the chin to resist the head flexion and extension, respectively (Figs. 101A, 101B).

In the sitting position, the therapist stands diagonally behind the patient with MCs similarly placed on the head and the chin. In this position, gravity equally resists both the flexion and the extension movements. With the head in a neutral position there is minimal influence of the tonic reflexes and righting reactions can be facilitated.

In P on E, the patterns can be performed with gravity assisting flexion and resisting extension (Figs. 101C, 101D).

The movement of rotation can be isolated in all of these postures. One contact is on the chin while the forearm of that hand resists on the side of the face (Figs. 101E, 101F).

Various techniques can be applied to these motions in the different postures. To improve stability or to gain range, RS can be performed. The MCs are placed to resist isometric contrac-

Neck patterns performed in P on E can enhance stability of shoulder and scapular muscles.

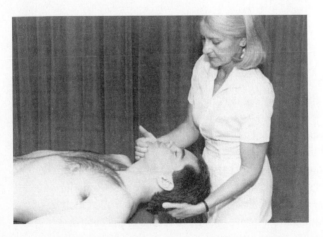

101A Neck flexion with L rotation—lengthened range.

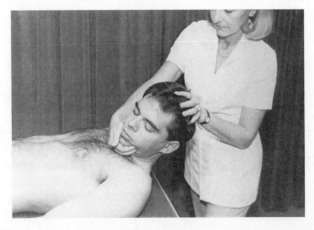

101B Neck flexion with L rotation—shortened range.

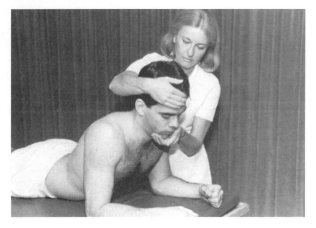

101C Neck flexion with L rotation—shortened range.

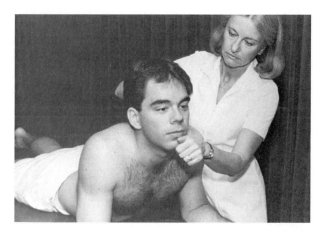

101D Neck extension with R rotation—mid range.

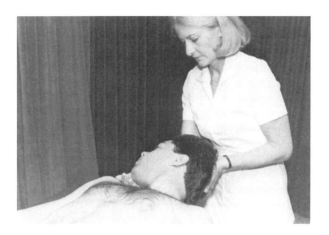

101E Neck rotation to R.

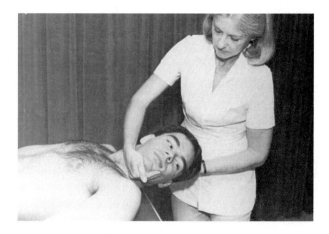

101F Neck rotation to L.

tions in opposite directions. HR is appropriate to gain ROM. The isometric submaximal contractions are usually performed to the agonist as contracting the antagonist in lengthened ranges may cause discomfort. SRH can be used to promote reversal movements.

Purpose/Treatment Goals

The purposes are to promote ROM in the head and the neck with the techniques of HR or RS; to enhance proximal stability (RS); and to facilitate smooth reversal of antagonists (SRH).

Head and neck patterns can be used to facilitate the reflex connection between the eyes and the head motions. Righting reactions that help to control automatic head movements can be promoted.

Patients with brainstem involvement frequently need improved control of these proximal areas. Improved head and neck stability and control is a primary goal for these patients.

For patients with neck pain and decreased cervical movement, these procedures are appropriate to increase ROM and decreased abnormal holding of cervical muscles. Following the gains in range promoted with HR and joint mobilization, stability and controlled mobility techniques are incorporated into the treatment to improve postural awareness and control.

When RS is applied in the P on E position, proximal stability of the upper trunk musculature can be indirectly promoted.

Problems with Application

In supine, neck flexion is resisted by gravity. The therapist may need to assist this motion if these muscles are not able to overcome gravitational effects. The therapist may resist all head and neck motions too vigorously. Care must be taken in all positions both with the amount of resistance and the amount of stretch. Excessive extension of the head and neck is avoided to prevent compromising of the vertebral artery and neural tissues.

Facial and Tongue Motions

Activity: Supine or sitting; facial and tongue motions
Technique: Slow reversal (SR), repeated contractions (RC), timing for emphasis (TE); MC as needed
Impairments: Facial muscle weakness; difficulty swallowing; dysarthria.

102

Description

Specific facial or tongue movements can be promoted in either supine or sitting. Use of a mirror will provide visual feedback that may enhance the response. Because most of the facial muscles are innervated bilaterally, promoting overflow from one side of the face to the other is usually successful. The facial muscles are primarily phasic and respond well to quick stretch and resistance. Techniques such as RC and TE that incorporate these two elements can be applied to most facial muscles with good results.

Tongue control progresses through the stages of control: mobility is the movement of the tongue in all directions, stability is the ability to groove the tongue or to suck, controlled mobility is proximal movement with the tip of the tongue stabilized (swallowing), and skill occurs with the distal part free to move (speech). Stretch and resisted movement can be provided to the tongue muscles with a moistened tongue depressor or a moistened gauze pad. To enhance movement of the soft palate a cotton swab can be used.

Lower Trunk Patterns

Activity: Supine; lower trunk flexion (LTF); knee flexion
Technique: Slow reversal hold (SRH); manual contacts on thighs, feet
Impairments: Weakness of lower trunk or lower extremities.

103

Description

The lower trunk patterns are named according to the direction of the movement, e.g., LTF to the left and the reverse movement of lower trunk extension (LTE) to the right. Similar to the upper trunk patterns, they combine asymmetrical extremity patterns. The pattern described is *LTF left* and *LTE right*. In this combination the R leg moves in the D1 pattern and the L leg in D2.

The patient is positioned near the edge of the plinth. The therapist stands by the LEs facing the patient. The patient is first guided through the movement to learn the pattern. During this passive movement the therapist's MCs are positioned under the thighs and the feet. The patient's hips, knees, and ankles are flexed to approximately 90 degrees in the direction of the L shoulder with

The pattern of lower trunk flexion combines lower extremity flexion with trunk flexion.

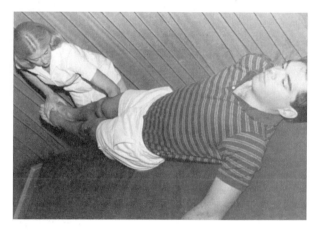

103A Lower trunk flexion initiation of movement.

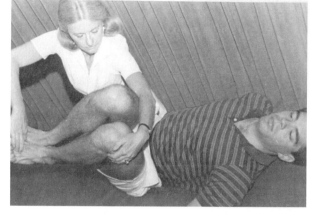

103B Lower trunk flexion shortened range.

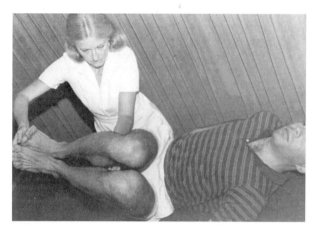

103C Lower trunk extension lengthened range.

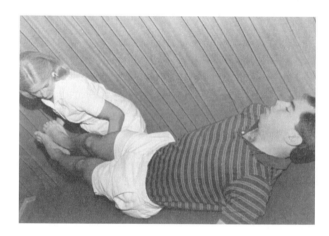

103D Lower trunk extension shortened range.

both the knees and the feet cross the midline. The legs are then moved into the extension pattern.

To begin resistance, the legs are positioned in extension. The distal MC is placed on the dorsum of the patient's feet to stretch the dorsiflexors; the proximal MC can be either on the anterior or posterior surface of the thighs (Fig. 103A). When placed on the anterior surface, stretch can be applied to the proximal muscles and resistance applied from the lengthened to the shortened range. If the proximal MC is on the posterior surface of the thigh, the therapist can more effectively add a traction force to the stretch and assist the patient during the initial ranges of trunk and hip flexion. This second method may be preferable for most patients. In the lengthened range of the flexor pattern, the lever arm is long as the hips and the knees begin the mass flexion pattern from the fully extended position. This initial flexion motion therefore may put a stress on the low back area, especially if the lower abdominals are weak. Thus, assistance may be needed as the legs flex against gravity. Approximately halfway through the range, when the pelvis is posteriorly tilted and the lever arm shorter, the proximal contact can be switched to the anterior surface of the thighs to provide resistance to the flexor muscles into their shortened range. The hold in the shortened range of flexion is applied with the proximal hand on the thighs resisting primarily trunk and hip activity while the distal hand resists the knee and the ankle (Fig. 103B).

To facilitate a smooth reversal of antagonists, the proximal hand maintains isometric resistance to the flexor pattern as the distal hand is shifted to the plantar surface of the feet with the thumb under the toes. With this distal placement, as well as with guidance from the proximal contact, the extensor pattern can be stretched in a diagonal direction toward the opposite (L) shoulder (Fig. 103C). After the patient responds to the stretch and verbal cues, and begins the extensor movement, the proximal hand is quickly positioned under the thighs to resist trunk and hip extension. The hold in the shortened range of extension combines an approximation force with resistance to the components of the pattern (Fig. 103D). The antagonistic movement or flexion is stretched again by moving the distal contact to the dorsum of the feet while the proximal hand maintains resistance to extension. Following the stretch, the pattern is resisted into the shortened range in the manner previously described. The reversals are repeated. During both movements the distal hand should be as distal as possible to facilitate the foot movement. Verbal commands may be "bring your legs up toward your opposite shoulder, hold it." "Push your legs down, turn your heels out toward me and hold."

Purpose/Treatment Goals

The purposes are to strengthen the lower trunk and lower extremity muscles; to improve the interaction of the two sides of the body; to facilitate a mass pattern in the lower extremities; and to promote overflow in the lower body area.

The trunk muscles that are primarily active during LTF to the left are the lower abdominal on the right and upper abdominal on the left. In the extensor phase, the lower back extensors are most active along with the gluteus medius in the R D1 leg and the gluteus maximus in the L D2 leg.

If the distal component is not innervated or very weak the MCs can be moved to the heels to provide support and resistance.

When this procedure is performed repetitively with minimal resistance it becomes an endurance training exercise for all the muscles participating in the movement.

Problems with Application

The therapist may not position the patient near enough to the edge of the plinth and thus have difficulty resisting the shortened range of flexion. The therapist may not be positioned close enough to the patient, which results in poor body mechanics particularly in the shortened range of extension. The resistance in this extensor range should be provided by the therapist's lower extremities, which flex with the patient's movement and not by the therapist's low back and upper extremities. Proper body mechanics, although always important, need special consideration with trunk procedures.

During the initiation of the flexor pattern the therapist observes the low back area to determine if the patient can maintain proper positioning. If an anterior tilt of the pelvis is evident, more assistance to the initial phase of the flexor motion may be needed.

The rotation, which occurs in the lower trunk and hips, should be initiated at the beginning of the movement so that in the shortened range of the flexor pattern the hips, knees, and feet are positioned across the midline. Care must be taken that the patient is correctly guided through the pattern.

Lower trunk flexion facilitates primarily lower abdominal and lower extremity muscles of the D1, D2 flexor patterns.

104

Activity: Supine; lower trunk flexion (LTF); knee flexion

Technique: Slow reversal hold (SRH) with timing for emphasis (TE); MC thighs/feet

Impairments: Weakness in abdominal, unilateral or bilateral lower extremity muscles; decreased interaction of left and right sides of body; decreased trunk rotation.

TE is used to elicit overflow effects from LE to trunk muscles.

Description

The lower trunk pattern is the same as just described. The technique of TE changes the focus of the procedure from general activation of the lower body musculature to strengthening of the lower abdominals when the flexor motion is emphasized. The technique of TE is appropriate if the patient has stronger musculature in the lower limbs than in the lower trunk. If such is the case overflow from the stronger LE muscles can be used to enhance the activity of the weaker abdominals.

To perform the procedure, the lower trunk flexor pattern is stretched and resisted until the hips, knees, and ankles are at 90 degrees of flexion. A strong isometric hold is performed to lock in these muscles. Focus then changes to the abdominals. With the limb flexors, primarily the hip flexors, "locked in," the quick stretch applied through the limbs will result in a stretch of the lower abdominals. The desired lower trunk movement facilitated by this stretch is curling or flexing and rotating one side of the pelvis off the plinth (Fig. 104A). This curling movement is resisted (TE). After a few repetitions, when the shortened range of trunk flexion with rotation is reached, an isometric hold is performed. The reversal extensor pattern is then stretched and resisted.

If the focus is on the extensor pattern, the LE extensors are resisted into their shortened range. In this range they are locked in with an isometric hold facilitated by approximation. The weaker low back extensors are then pivoted (TE).

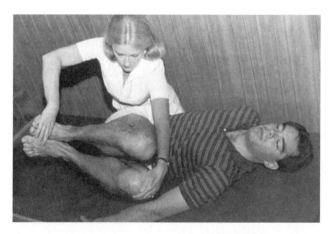

104A Lower trunk flexion—TE abdominals.

Purpose/Treatment Goals

The purpose is to strengthen the lower abdominals or the lower back extensors. Just as the upper trunk muscles are facilitated by upper trunk patterns, the lower abdominal and back extensors are facilitated by lower trunk patterns.

The lower abdominals flex the lower trunk against gravity, therefore the amount of resistance provided has to be carefully monitored. Because the back extensors are assisted by gravity, resistance must be sufficient to resist the contraction. In either instance, TE, which promotes a maximum effort, should be repeated only a few times in one treatment session.

For the many patients with lower abdominal weakness, this procedure, if correctly applied, can be beneficial. If, because of extreme weakness in the abdominals or tightness in the hip flexors, the pelvis anteriorly tilts in the beginning of the range, the patient can be positioned in the shortened range of LTF before TE is applied. If tightness in the lower back area exists and interferes with range into lower trunk flexion, the range limitations need to be addressed before attempting to strengthen the lower abdominals. LTF can be performed independently by beginning in hooklying and bringing the knees toward one shoulder while maintaining a neutral pelvic and low back position.

Problems with Application

Therapists may have difficulty locking in the hip flexors and actually applying the stretch to the trunk. Instead, the stretch frequently is incorrectly applied to the hip flexors. If the hold in the shortened range of hip flexion can be maintained, the technique of TE should be correctly performed.

Lower trunk extension facilitates primarily lower trunk extensors and lower extremity muscles of the D1, D2 extensor patterns.

Activity: Supine; lower trunk flexion (LTF), knee flexion
Technique: Hold relax (HR); MC pelvis and thigh
Impairments: Decreased mobility of low back extensors.

105

Description

The activity of LTF is the same as in the previous procedures. The technique of HR is applied in the shortened range of LTF to increase the extensibility of the low back extensors. Because the shortened range is being emphasized, the therapist stands in the diagonal in the shortened range of the flexor pattern. MCs are placed on the pelvis and thigh and the therapist's body, shoulder, may be used to apply resistance (Fig. 105A). Isometric resistance can be applied to either the abdominals (agonist) or the back extensors (antagonist). If the abdominals are resisted, strengthening of these muscles occurs along with reciprocal inhibition of the back extensors. Relaxation follows the isometric contraction and trunk flexion with rotation is minimally resisted into the newly gained range. During this movement the pelvis should rise off the plinth; an increase in the hip flexion range should not occur. The technique is repeated until no additional gain in LTF occurs. Verbal commands may be "bring your knees up to your opposite shoulder, hold it, relax and let me support your legs, now bring your legs up further and curl your pelvis up." Isometric contraction of the extensors can also be performed but is more difficult to control and may not be as successful.

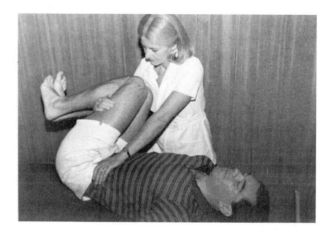

105A Lower trunk flexion.

Purpose/Treatment Goals

HR with LTF can increase extensibility of trunk extensors.

The purpose is to increase the extensibility of the low back extensors, especially the quadratus lumborum.

If the patient cannot tolerate the amount of lower body motion that occurs with this procedure performed in supine, sidelying with forward pelvic rotation or lateral trunk elongation may be substituted. In sidelying, the therapist can emphasize gross lower trunk flexion with rotation motion or specifically facilitate intersegmental vertebral motion.

Problem with Application

Therapist may inappropriately emphasize the hip motion and not the pelvic and lower trunk motion.

Bilateral Lower Extremity Patterns

106

Activity: Supine; bilateral symmetrical (BS) D2E, knees straight
Technique: Slow reversal hold (SRH), shortened range of emphasis (SE); MC heels
Impairments: Weakness in lower trunk extensors or gluteus maximus; weakness in pelvic floor muscles.

Description

In a treatment progression, bilateral patterns usually follow the trunk patterns. The patient is in supine with the heels or lower legs extended off the edge of the plinth. The therapist stands at the foot of the plinth facing the patient. The patient's legs are positioned in BS D2E, that combines hip extension, adduction and external rotation, knee extension, and foot plantarflexion with inversion. The therapist's MCs are positioned on the heels with fingers together on the medial surface and thumbs on the lateral surface. The patient is first passively moved through partial range of the D2F pattern to experience the feeling of the movement: hip flexion, abduction and internal rotation, knee extension, and ankle dorsiflexion with eversion. The knees remain extended throughout movement into both directions. During the flexion motion the therapist's

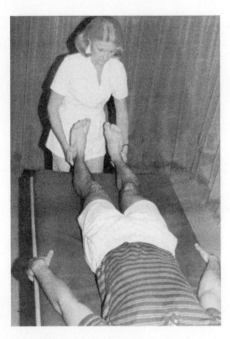
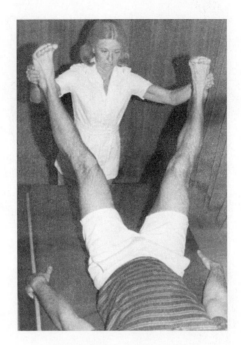

106A BS D2F—lengthened range.

106B B2 D2F—shortened range.

MCs pivot around the heel, so that in the shortened range of hip flexion the thumbs are on the medial surface and the fingers on the lateral surface of the heel. Although the MCs can be placed more distally on the foot, the patient's limb movements can be controlled more easily with the MCs on the heels. During the extension pattern, the therapist's MCs pivot around the heel to the original placement.

To resist the activity, the legs are positioned in extension and the flexor pattern is stretched (Fig. 106A). Because the legs are in contact with the plinth, the stretch is primarily to the hip's rotational component in combination with traction. The lever arm is long during the initial phase of the flexor movement. Assistance, therefore, must be provided to the flexion pattern until the mid range is approached. During the flexion pattern the therapist's contacts pivot around the heel as described. In the mid to shortened range of the flexion pattern a minimal holding contraction can be applied (Fig. 106B). A stretch is then applied to the extensors (Fig. 106C), followed by resistance through the range until the patient reaches the shortened range of extension (Fig. 106D). At this point, an isometric contraction of the extensors, adductors, and external rotators is resisted.

BS D2E facilitates lower trunk extensors and lower extremity extensors and adductors.

The focus of this procedure is usually on the shortened range of the extensor pattern as this is the range in which the extensors optimally function. To promote a holding contraction in this shortened range, an approximation force is added.

Purpose/Treatment Goals

The purposes are to enhance isometric holding in the shortened range of D2E and to strengthen the gluteus maximus, the adductors and the pelvic floor muscles in the extension phase.

Resistance to hip extension with adduction facilitates holding of pelvic floor musculature.

This procedure is appropriate for patients with urinary incontinence and/or weakness in the pubococcygeal muscle. This problem is common in elderly patients or multiparous women. As the patient is holding in the shortened range of D2E, tightening of the pelvic floor muscles can be enhanced.

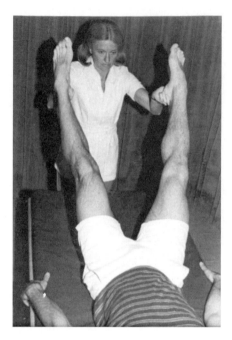

106C BS D2E—lengthened range.

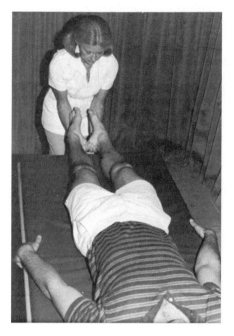

106D BS D2E—shortened range.

Problems with Application

Therapists may give too much resistance during the flexion phase causing the pelvis to tilt anteriorly. If excessive tilting occurs the flexion motion must be assisted. Therapists may lose control of the movement if the patient is allowed to move through full ROM of straight leg raising (SLR). Because the focus of the procedure is primarily on the extension pattern, movement into the shortened range of flexion is unnecessary.

107

Activity: Supine; bilateral symmetrical (BS) D1E, knees straight

Technique: Slow reversal hold (SRH) with timing for emphasis (TE) to hip extension; MC heels

Impairments: Weakness of gluteus medius and trunk extensors.

Description

The patient is supine with the lower legs partially extended off the edge of the plinth. The therapist stands at the foot of the plinth facing the patient. The patient's LEs are positioned in D1E, that combines hip extension, abduction, and internal rotation, knee extension, and ankle plantarflexion with eversion. MCs are placed with the thumbs on the lateral surface of the heels and the fingers on the medial surface. The patient is passively moved into the mid range of the flexor motion, that combines hip flexion, adduction, and external rotation, knee extension, and ankle dorsiflexion with inversion. The two directions of the pattern are repeated. The knee remains in extension throughout the movement in both directions. For both the flexor and the extensor phases of D1 the MCs remain on the heels with the thumb on the lateral surface of the heel.

To resist the activity, the legs are positioned in extension. The flexor pattern is stretched

.

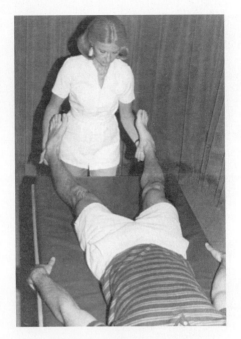

107A BS D1F—lengthened range.

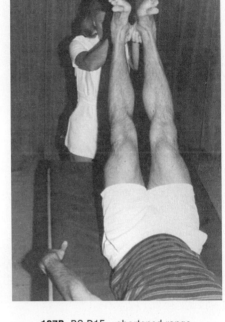

107B BS D1F—shortened range.

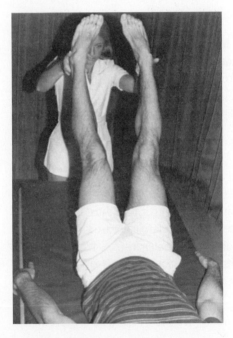

107C BS D1E—lengthened range.

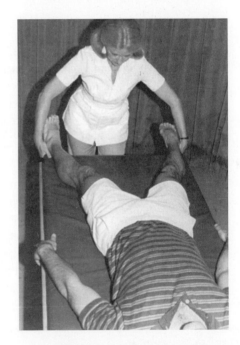

107D BS D1E—shortened range.

with a traction, rotation, and abduction motion (Fig. 107A). Because the limbs are in contact with the plinth, stretch into extension is limited. As with the D2 pattern, assistance may be needed during the initial phase of flexion if the pelvis tends to tilt anteriorly. In the mid to shortened range of D1F (flexion, adduction, external rotation), a slight hold can be applied (Fig. 107B), followed by stretch to the components of the extensor pattern (Fig. 107C). The patient is then guided and resisted into the diagonal extensor movement (Fig. 107D). Resistance can be applied throughout the extension pattern but emphasis is in the shortened range of extension.

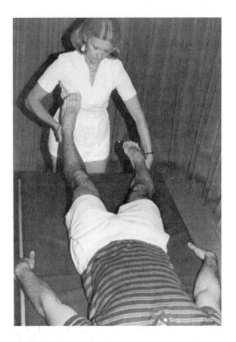

107E BS D1E; TE RLE.

To perform the technique of TE, the stronger leg is resisted into the shortened range of D1E where approximation facilitates the isometric contraction. This leg is "locked in" and resistance maintained as the weaker leg is pivoted, i.e., repeated contractions are applied to the leg as it moves into the shortened range of D1E (Fig. 107E). When the shortened range is achieved, isometric resistance is applied to both legs.

BS D1E facilitates lower trunk extensors and lower extremity extensors and abductors.

Purpose/Treatment Goals

The purpose is to strengthen the gluteus medius and trunk extensors.

Because hip extension is assisted by gravity, sufficient manual resistance must be applied. To promote overflow from the stronger to the weaker limb, the stronger limb must be "locked in" with an isometric contraction as the weaker limb is being pivoted, or emphasized.

Bilateral abduction occurs in the pattern; Raimiste's phenomenon (resisted abduction of one limb facilitates abduction of the other) may facilitate the response of the weaker limb.

Although not described, TE can be applied in a similar manner to the D2 pattern when strengthening the gluteus maximus is the goal.

Problems with Application

Movement occurs in a diagonal line and not in a circular direction. The patient may tend to "windmill" or move in a circular motion rather than in the diagonal or groove of the pattern. The therapist must guide the patient into the correct direction of movement, especially during extension.

Both the D1 and D2 patterns are performed in a symmetrical combination. With many people, however, reinforcement occurs reciprocally in the lower extremities. In such cases, the stronger leg, which is locked in during TE, will tend to drift into flexion. If this occurs, another activity, such as lower trunk extension or a unilateral D1E pattern, which does not require symmetrical reinforcement, should be substituted. Unilateral patterns should also be used if the therapist observes knee hyperextension occurring during the performance of BS D1 or D2 activities. Manual contacts in lower trunk extensor and unilateral patterns can provide support and resistance to the knee as needed.

Other combinations, such as asymmetrical and reciprocal straight leg patterns, may be included in treatment but are difficult for the therapist to control and for the patient to perform in the supine position.

Emphasis on the knee musculature can be accomplished in both prone and sitting.

108

Activity: Prone; bilateral asymmetrical (BA), flexion/extension
Technique: Slow reversal hold (SRH), hold relax active movement (HRAM), hold relax (HR), agonistic reversals (AR); MC feet
Impairments: Marked weakness of quadriceps; decreased hamstring control; decreased knee mobility in flexion or extension.

Description

The patient is prone with feet over the edge of the plinth which is padded under the ankles. Some patients may need extra padding under the thigh if the patella is painful. The therapist stands at the foot of the plinth in the direction of the diagonal pattern to be performed. The patient is moved passively through the pattern of asymmetrical knee flexion to the right, extension to the left. As the knees flex, the ankles plantarflex and as the knees extend, the feet dorsiflex in an advanced combination.

To resist the procedure, the patient's knees are positioned in extension. The therapist's thumbs are distally placed on the plantar surface of the feet and a stretch is applied to the plantarflexors and knee flexors (Fig. 108A). As the patient moves into knee flexion the therapist places the fingers on the plantar surface of the feet. A hold is performed at approximately 90 degrees of knee flexion (Fig. 108B). To facilitate the antagonist pattern and to stretch the knee ex-

In prone, the hamstrings contract against manual and gravitational resistance. Quadriceps are assisted by gravity.

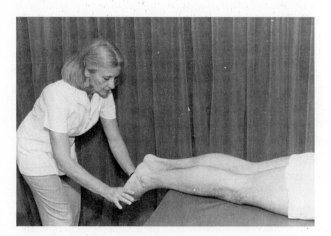

108A Asymmetrical knee flexion—lengthened range.

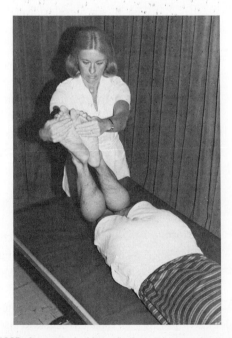

108B Asymmetrical knee flexion—shortened range.

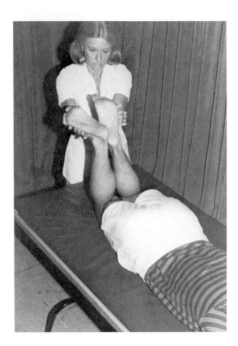

108C Asymmetrical knee extension—lengthened range.

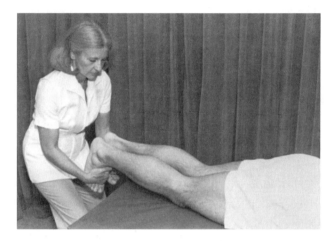

108D Asymmetrical knee extension—shortened range.

tensors and dorsiflexors, the heels of the therapist's hands are placed on the dorsiflexor surface (Fig. 108C). As the movement into knee extension occurs, the therapist's hands pivot around the foot and the forearms supinate so that the fingers are on the dorsiflexor surface to resist into the shortened range of the pattern (Fig. 108D).

To summarize the placement of MCs, knee flexion and ankle plantarflexion are stretched with the thumbs, then the fingers are placed on the balls of the feet to resist those motions. To reverse direction, the heels of the hands are positioned on the dorsum of the feet to stretch ankle dorsiflexion and knee extension, then the hands and forearms pivot so that resistance is provided by the fingers on the dorsiflexor surface.

Many patients in prone will have difficulty interpreting up and down or right and left commands. Verbal commands must be kept simple and as easy as possible to follow. For example, "point your toes up toward the ceiling, and bend your knees." "Bring your toes and ankles down toward the floor and straighten your knees."

The technique of HRAM is appropriate if the patient has difficulty initiating knee flexion from the lengthened range. A hold in the shortened range of knee flexion, at about 90 degrees, is followed by relaxation and quick passive movement into the lengthened range. A quick stretch is then applied to the hamstrings followed by tracking resistance to the isotonic flexion contraction. To further enhance the contraction of the knee flexors, RC can be superimposed. The lengthened range of the hamstrings is emphasized as this is the range in which they most frequently function, particularly during ambulation.

AR will enhance eccentric control of the hamstrings that is needed during the latter part of the swing phase of gait. This technique begins with a concentric contraction from the lengthened to the shortened range of knee flexion as described. In the shortened range, the verbal command "make it difficult for me to pull your legs down" or "let your legs down slowly" is given. The eccentric contraction of the hamstrings is resisted into the lengthened range. If the patient begins to lose control (the contraction is not smooth) near the lengthened range of knee flexion, the movement is reversed to the concentric contraction back into the shortened range. The goal of the procedure is for the patient to control an eccentric contraction throughout the

full range. Because the hamstrings lose their biomechanical advantage in the lengthened range, eccentric control in this range is frequently problematic. AR is performed usually through increments of range emphasizing control in the lengthened range. As only one direction of the pattern is performed, MCs remain on the plantar surface of the feet.

Purpose/Treatment Goals

The purposes are to facilitate mobility, ROM (HR), and the initiation of movement, of the hamstrings (HRAM); to increase stability of the quadriceps (SHRC); to promote a smooth reversal of antagonists (SRH); to enhance eccentric control of the hamstrings (AR).

In prone quadriceps can be emphasized in shortened ranges and hamstrings in lengthened ranges.

In this activity the technique of HR can be performed to increase range into either knee flexion or extension. Increased extensibility of the rectus femoris, which is stretched over both the hip and the knee, can be easily accomplished with the technique of HR applied to the agonist. However, because the hamstrings are in a position of active insufficiency during knee flexion, only minimal resistance can be applied during the isometric contraction. The isometric contraction is not applied to the antagonistic quadriceps in this lengthened range, as both the active plus passive tension may cause muscle tearing. Also, the knee extensors are on prolonged stretch and may be inhibited if an isometric contraction is applied to the extensors in this range. Elongation, not inhibition is the goal. The isometric hold is judiciously applied to the hamstrings followed by relaxation and further active range into knee flexion. ROM into knee extension also can be accomplished with HR.

During the performance of the bilateral patterns the legs are kept in contact with each other to improve the sensory feedback and enhance overflow from one limb to the other. Although this activity is usually performed to improve hamstring functioning, quadriceps that are below a fair muscle grade can be strengthened in shortened ranges with this bilateral prone pattern. Both quadriceps and hamstring control are important for knee stability and must be maximized in those patients lacking ligamentous stability.

Problems with Application

Placement of MCs in this procedure may be difficult for some therapists to learn. Before resistance is added, the therapist should practice changing MCs during the reversal movements.

Because the hamstrings move into a position of active insufficiency during flexion, the extremely shortened range should be avoided to prevent muscle cramping. Also, the rectus femoris is in a position of passive insufficiency during the shortened range of flexion and may be overstretched.

Some patients may have a great deal of difficulty performing the advanced movement combination of knee extension with ankle dorsiflexion or knee flexion with plantarflexion. In such cases, a mass pattern can be performed allowing knee flexion with ankle dorsiflexion and knee extension with plantarflexion. However, because this combination is more difficult for the therapist to control and does not promote the advanced combinations needed for gait, the pattern explained above is preferable.

109

Activity: Sitting; bilateral symmetrical (BS) D1

Technique: Slow reversal hold (SRH) with timing for emphasis (TE); MC feet

Impairments: Difficulty reversing movements; weakness in quadriceps or hamstrings; weakness or abnormal timing of distal segments.

Description

The emphasis of this procedure, similar to the preceding one, is on the knee and the ankle musculature. The patient is short sitting on a plinth. The patient's UEs can hold onto the plinth for support and to provide overflow. The therapist is facing the patient with feet in stride to enlarge the BoS. The subject's legs are in BS D1E with the legs positioned in abduction and internal rotation, knee flexion, and ankle plantarflexion with eversion. The direction of the pattern is described for the *hip* component and not the intermediate knee joint. The antagonistic pattern is BS D1F with hip adduction and external rotation, knee extension, and ankle dorsiflexion and inversion. During the performance of the pattern the distal component should lead the movement to promote normal timing. Prior to adding resistance the therapist moves the patient through the pattern to teach the movement.

To resist the activity, the legs are positioned with the knees flexed. The therapist's MCs are placed distally on the dorsiflexor surface; the thumbs are medial and the fingers lateral (Fig. 109A). The quadriceps, dorsiflexors, and invertors are stretched and resisted into the shortened range. Most of the resistance is provided by the web space of the therapist's hand (Fig. 109B). As the patient extends the knee into D1F, the MCs can be maintained or rotated around the feet so that the fingers are facing medially rather than laterally (Fig. 109C). This change of MCs allows the therapist to have better control of inversion and rotation. A hold is given in the shortened range, which combines resistance to both the foot and the knee components. To stretch the antagonistic pattern the MCs slide around the lateral side of the foot onto the plantar surface (Fig. 109D). Stretch, then resistance, is applied to the hamstrings, plantarflexors, and evertors

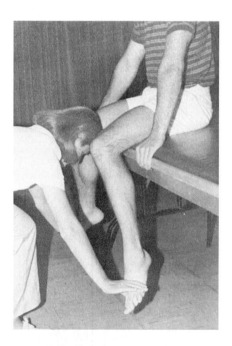

109A BS D1F—lengthened range.

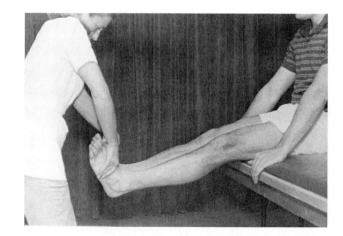

109B BS D1F—shortened range.

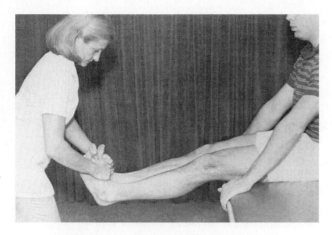

109C BS D1F—shortened range; alternate contacts.

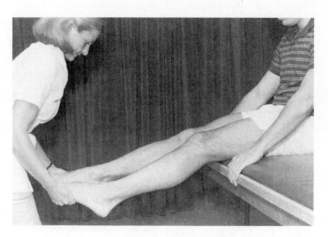

109D BS D1E—lengthened range.

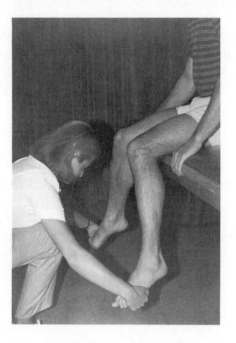

109E BS D1E—shortened range.

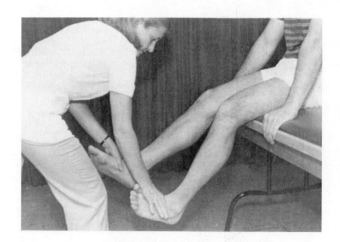

109F BS D1F; TE L quadriceps.

moving into the shortened range of D1E where a hold is resisted (Fig. 109E). The reversal is initiated by moving the MCs back to the dorsiflexor surface of the feet where stretch is applied and the sequence repeated.

The technique of TE applied to bilateral patterns is appropriate when there is an imbalance of strength. For example, a patient may have weak quadriceps on the left. Using this BS pattern the quadriceps on the right can be isometrically resisted to promote overflow to the left. Because the quadriceps muscle is an extensor, "locking in" is performed near the shortened range, avoiding complete extension and biomechanical locking of the knee. The procedure begins with both legs in D1E with the knees flexed. Stretch and resistance are applied to both legs. Because the left quadriceps is weaker it may not move through the complete range. The right quadriceps is locked in near the shortened range performing a strong isometric contraction. The left quadriceps response is then enhanced with repeated contractions (Fig. 109F). When the left leg reaches full extension, isometric resistance is applied to both legs before the antagonistic pat-

In sitting the quadriceps contract against gravitational and manual resistance. Hamstrings are assisted by gravity.

tern is bilaterally stretched and resisted. Because the weak muscle is an extensor, resistance is initially emphasized in the shortened range to minimize possible inhibition. As the quadriceps increase in strength, resistance can be provided in more lengthened ranges.

TE also can be performed to the knee flexors. Stretch and resistance is applied bilaterally to D1E with knee flexion. The hamstrings of the stronger leg are resisted to approximately 90 degrees, where they can hold most strongly. RC are then performed on the weak knee flexors emphasizing the lengthened range important for ambulation.

Purpose/Treatment Goals

In sitting quadriceps can be emphasized in shortened ranges and hamstrings in lengthened ranges.

The purposes are to promote a smooth reversal of antagonistic movements (SRH); to strengthen the quadriceps or hamstrings (TE); and to promote the advanced movement combinations of dorsiflexion with knee extension and plantar flexion with knee flexion.

The vastus medialis seems to be more active during D1F than during D2F. For those patients who exhibit a laterally tracking patella during knee extension, strengthening of this portion of the quadriceps may be indicated and may be enhanced with this pattern as well as with weight bearing activities. Although manual resistance and assistance can be varied, these sitting patterns are most appropriate for quadriceps that have a 3/5 grade or above (gravity resists) or for hamstrings with a 3/5 grade or below (gravity assists). Because the hamstrings are stretched at the hip by virtue of the position, external stretch added by the therapist can easily facilitate a flexor response.

Problems with Application

Therapists may have difficulty with the reversal of MCs and should practice the change of contacts before adding any resistance. The therapist's feet must be in stride to afford a large BoS and promote proper body mechanics. A healthy person playing the role of a patient should pretend to be weak in the muscles being emphasized to give the therapist a better feel of what will occur clinically as well as to protect his/her own muscles from excessive amounts of resistance.

110

Activity: Sitting; bilateral symmetrical D2
Technique: Slow reversal hold (SRH) with timing for emphasis (TE); MC feet
Impairments: Difficulty reversing movements; weakness in quadriceps or hamstrings; weakness or abnormal timing of distal segments.

Description

The patient is short sitting holding onto the plinth. The therapist with feet in stride faces the patient. In the D2E pattern, the hips are adducted and slightly externally rotated, the knees flexed and the feet together in plantarflexion and inversion. The D2F motion combines hip abduction and internal rotation, knee extension with dorsiflexion and eversion.

Resistance to the pattern begins with the legs in D2E and the knees flexed. The therapist's MCs are on the dorsiflexor and evertor surface of the feet with the fingers lateral and the thumbs medial (Fig. 110A). Stretch, then resistance, is applied to ankle dorsiflexion with eversion and knee extension (Fig. 110B). In the shortened range of D2F, an isometric contraction is resisted then the hands slide around the lateral aspect of the feet and onto the plantar surface to stretch and resist the antagonistic D2E pattern of plantarflexion, inversion, and knee flexion (Figs. 110C, 110D).

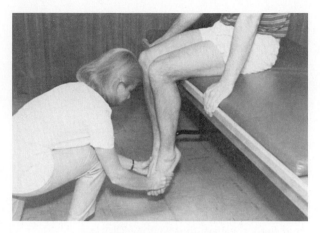

110A D2F—lengthened range.

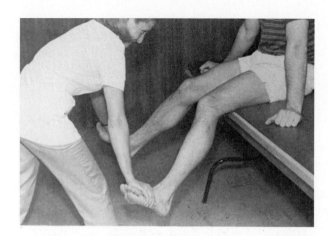

110B D2F—shortened range.

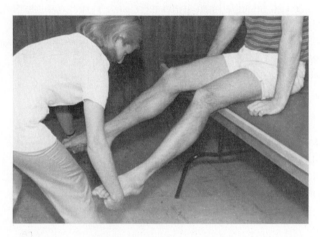

110C D2E—lengthened range.

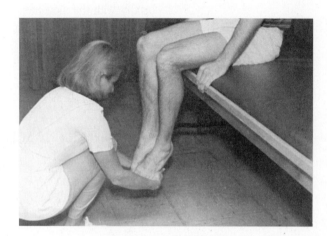

110D D2E—shortened range.

TE can be applied to either the quadriceps or hamstrings in a similar manner to that performed in the D1 pattern described earlier.

Purpose/Treatment Goals

The purposes are to promote a smooth reversal of antagonists; to strengthen the hamstrings or lateral portion of the quadriceps; and to promote dorsiflexion with eversion combined with knee extension.

For many patients with central nervous system dysfunction, the combination of dorsiflexion with eversion and knee extension is important to promote the functional movements needed during ambulation.

For those patients with a lateral sprain of the ankle strengthening dorsiflexion with eversion is an important aspect of rehabilitation.

111

Activity: Sitting; bilateral reciprocal (BR) D1, D2

Technique: Slow reversal hold (SRH), timing for emphasis (TE); MC feet

Impairments: Weak quadriceps or hamstrings.

Description

Strong quadriceps can be used to facilitate weak contralateral hamstrings.

The patient's position remains the same as in the symmetrical patterns. The therapist faces the patient. To best control the patient's LE movements during these patterns, the therapist's feet move forward and backward in a reciprocal manner in time with the patient's movement (Figs. 111A, 111B). To familiarize the patient with the hip, knee, and ankle movements, the patient is moved first through the symmetrical pattern. From the symmetrical position one leg is reversed, i.e., moved into flexion, and the reciprocal pattern then rhythmically reversed. The passive movements are performed slowly, then, as both the patient and the therapist become comfortable with the movement, resistance can be added and speed increased. Verbal commands are simply "switch" or "change." MCs on the feet are reciprocally altered from the anterior to the plantar surfaces.

The technique of TE is performed in a similar manner to that described in the symmetrical patterns. The patient now reinforces reciprocally, for example, the extensors of one leg can be used to enhance the flexor response of the other leg.

Purpose/Treatment Goals

Reciprocal patterns promote movements needed for gait.

The purpose is to promote a smooth reversal of antagonists in a functional reciprocal pattern. Because most people reinforce reciprocally in the lower extremities, this pattern makes use of normal neurophysiological and neuroanatomical connections as well as the natural combination that occurs during ambulation.

Problems with Application

Many therapists have difficulty coordinating their MCs and controlling the patient's reciprocal movements. Attempts are often made by the therapist to perform the patterns with no foot or body movement. The therapist must practice to achieve the coordination required for these very

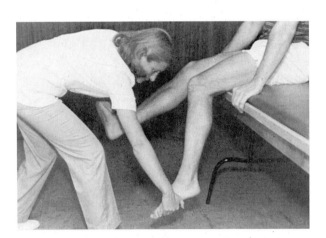

111A Reciprocal D1—L hamstrings, R quadriceps.

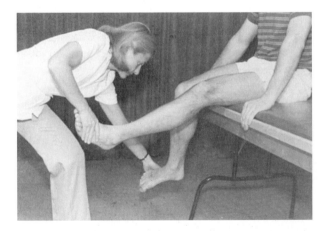

111B Reciprocal D1—L quadriceps, R hamstrings.

valuable and functional patterns. It is often more difficult for the therapist to learn these patterns than for the patient to perform them.

In a sitting position, bilateral asymmetrical and cross-diagonal patterns also can be performed. These patterns use different combinations of reinforcement than those just described and thus can promote overflow from other muscles groups.

Unilateral Lower Extremity Patterns

Activity: Sitting; unilateral D1, D2
Technique: Hold relax (HR), rhythmic stabilization (RS), contract relax (CR); MC foot
Impairments: Decreased mobility (ROM) into knee flexion or extension; decreased muscle stability.

112

Description

All three of these techniques can be used in either the D1 or D2 pattern to gain mobility–ROM by increasing the extensibility of the contractile tissues. This procedure is appropriate for patients demonstrating decreased passive ROM due to muscle tightness. For many patients with limitation in both extension and flexion, range into knee extension and improving the strength of the quadriceps are the initial goals. As the knee is resisted into extension, the quadriceps, the agonist, are strengthened and the hamstrings, the antagonist, are reciprocally inhibited.

To perform HR, both of the therapist's MCs are on the foot, one on the heel and the other on the forefoot. The knee is actively extended to the point of limitation in either of the diagonal directions (Fig. 112A). With both MCs applying pressure toward flexion a moderate level of isometric tension is slowly developed in the quadriceps. The therapist then alters manual contacts to support the leg and relaxation is allowed. Active movement into the new range is then resisted to tolerance. The technique is reapplied until no additional range into knee extension can be gained. During the holding portion of the HR technique only moderate isometric resistance is applied as too much resistance may inhibit the quadriceps or cause pain. Because pain may be a symptom during early stages of rehabilitation, relaxation may be difficult for the patient and adequate time should be allowed. The verbal commands are "hold, don't let me move your leg," or "don't let me push your leg down." The therapist does not say "push against me" as too much tension may result in pain or even injury to a weakened muscle.

When knee extension is the goal, the quadriceps are the agonist.

When increased range into knee flexion is the goal, the hamstrings are the agonist and the quadriceps the antagonist. Range into knee flexion or relaxation of the quadriceps can be achieved in a similar manner as just described. At the point of limitation into flexion a gradual isometric contraction of the hamstrings is resisted (Fig. 112B). The verbal command is "hold, don't let me straighten your knee," followed by relaxation and movement into more knee flexion.

In both of these procedures the isometric contraction is applied to the agonistic muscle. Although in HR the isometric contraction also can be applied directly to the tight antagonistic muscle, isometric resistance to the agonist is preferred. With this method, contraction of the agonist is enhanced while the antagonist is simultaneously inhibited. The agonist contraction also actively glides the bony components of the knee joint in the correct direction for the subsequent movement. In addition, the manual resistance into the pain-free or nonlimited range may be less anxiety producing for the patient. To increase range into knee flexion the therapist should avoid resisting the antagonistic quadriceps in their lengthened range, especially during early phases of treatment. In early stages of rehabilitation the quadriceps may be weak. If it is isometrically

When knee flexion is the goal, the hamstrings are the agonist.

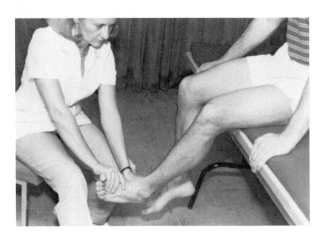

112A D1F, Knee extending; HR to quadriceps.

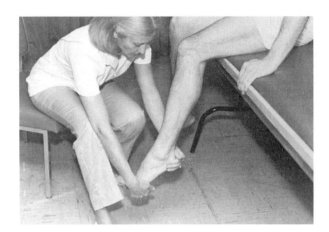

112B D1E, knee flexing; HR to hamstrings.

resisted in lengthened ranges excessive inhibition may occur making subsequent full active knee extension difficult to attain.

HR can be applied in either the D1 or D2 pattern depending on which motions are limited. For example, if knee extension and tibial external rotation are desired, then movement into the D1 flexor pattern may be more appropriate. If the lateral quadriceps muscle appears to be tighter than the medial portion of the quadriceps, then movement into the D2E knee flexion pattern may be the better choice.

RS is another technique incorporating primarily isometric contractions, that can be used to increase ROM. A simultaneous goal achieved with RS can be an increase in the muscular stability around the knee. To begin the technique both MCs are placed on the patient's foot, one on the heel and one on the forefoot. Although both contacts resist all components, the heel contact emphasizes primarily tibial rotation and the forefoot contact emphasizes primarily knee flexion and extension.

To increase range into knee extension in either the D1 or D2 pattern with RS, the therapist minimally resists the agonistic muscle, the quadriceps, to the point of limitation. In that range both MCs resist an isometric contraction of the agonistic dorsiflexor and quadriceps. The MC on the heel alters resistance to the antagonistic pattern so that resistance is being given simultaneously in opposite directions promoting contraction of both quadriceps and hamstrings (Fig. 112C). These opposite resistive forces are rhythmically altered a few times before isometric resistance is applied again with both MCs to the agonist followed by active resisted movement into more knee extension. At the new point of limitation the technique is reapplied. During the alteration of resistive forces the component that seems to require the most verbal cueing is the tibial rotation, which is primarily resisted by the MC on the heel. The verbal command might be "don't let me turn your heel in, now don't let me turn it out." The other components of flexion and extension resisted primarily by the MC on the forefoot do not seem to require as much verbal direction.

CR is the most strenuous of the three techniques that can be used to increase range in contractile tissues. Unlike the technique of HR, CR appears to be most effective when directly applied to the tight antagonistic muscle. CR involves an immediate and maximal buildup of muscle tension and active movement of the rotational component. For example, if the knee is limited into extension by tight hamstrings, the knee is extended to the point of limitation in either the D1 or D2 pattern. MCs are placed on the heel and on the plantar surface on the forefoot. With vigorous verbal commands the therapist asks the patient to bend the knee and turn the foot either in or out depending on the diagonal chosen (tibial rotation). The knee flexion component is isometrically resisted but the rotational component is allowed to move isotonically (Figs. 112D,

Resistance is graded with HR, RS. No joint movement is allowed.

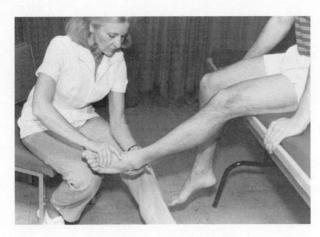

112C D1F, knee extending; RS.

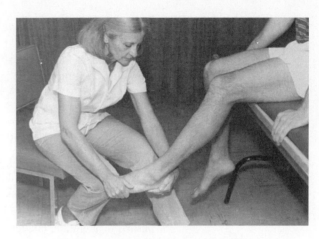

112D D1E, knee flexing; CR to hamstrings.

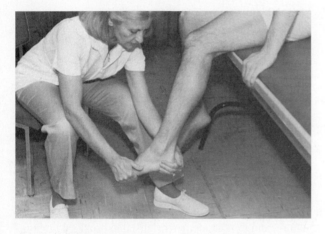

112E D1E, knee flexing; CR to hamstrings.

112E). When the rotational component is completed, relaxation occurs and active, minimally resisted movement into knee extension is encouraged. In this new range the technique is reapplied. CR is not usually applied to the quadriceps for the reasons stated earlier and is never used when pain is a factor.

Resistance is maximal with CR. Only the rotational component is allowed to move through range.

Purpose/Treatment Goals

The purpose is to increase range of the contractile tissues of the knee in a patient with musculoskeletal dysfunction. Although HR can be applied to either the agonist or the antagonist, it is most appropriately applied to the agonist. HR as described was applied to the diagonal patterns to specifically decrease muscular limitations. However, if rotatory stresses are contraindicated, e.g., patients with ligamentous strains or who have undergone surgical reconstruction, HR can be applied in a straight plane. For patients such as those with total knee replacements, knee flexion rather than extension may be the first goal to be accomplished.

RS may be more difficult to apply but is effective both in increasing range and in promoting muscular stability. RS also can be applied to promote the goals of improved stability at the ankle and foot.

CR appears to be most effective when applied to a tight muscle that functions as a flexor and that has a large rotary component (e.g., the hamstrings). *CR should never be used when pain is a factor.*

All of these techniques should be used in conjunction with soft tissue and joint mobilization procedures and thermal modalities when tightness exists in both the contractile as well as the noncontractile tissues.

Problems with Application

The use of proper verbal commands is essential to the success of these techniques. To promote an isometric contraction with HR and RS, the verbal command is "hold, don't let me move you." When isometric contractions are desired, the command to "push" is not used. The therapist should control the amount of tension developed in the muscle and this is most easily accomplished by a gradual buildup of isometric tension. If an isotonic contraction is involved as with CR, "turn and push" or "pull" are appropriate. The coordination of the verbal commands and MCs associated with RS can be difficult for some therapists. Proceed slowly with the three procedures until the differences in application and indications for use are clear.

113

Activity: Sitting; unilateral D1 or D2 patterns

Technique: Slow reversal (SR) or normal timing (NT); MC heel and forefoot

Impairments: Difficulty with sequencing, timing and reversing of knee and ankle movements.

Description

In the sitting position, unilateral LE patterns can be performed to enhance the smooth reversal of antagonistic knee and ankle musculature, and to promote normal distal to proximal timing of movement.

With the patient in short sitting, the therapist places MCs on the heel and forefoot of one leg to resist the pattern. In the D1F pattern the medial quadriceps is combined with dorsiflexion and inversion, and in the D2F pattern the lateral quadriceps with dorsiflexion and eversion. As with the previous procedure, in sitting the contact on the heel primarily resists tibial rotation and the contact on the forefoot resists the flexion and extension components at both the knee and the ankle. During the technique of SR the speed of the reversing movements can be increased until the patient can perform quick reversals of antagonists. With the technique of NT, the movement of the distal foot and ankle components is encouraged by repeated stretches before the knee is allowed to move through range.

Purpose/Treatment Goals

The purpose is to promote quick reversal of the knee muscles and the normal timing of movement in an advanced combination. These are advanced goals for many patients with orthopedic and central nervous system dysfunction. In these procedures the emphasis is on the skill stage of movement control and promoting coordinated timing and sequencing of movement. The assumption is made that the patient has the strength to move through the pattern and that the preceding stages of control have been achieved.

During the performance of these movements, a general rule is that the therapist's distal contact remains distal. As the patterns are reversed the more distal contact always moves to the opposite surface before the proximal contact is changed. This sequencing is to prevent the relaxation during the reversal of antagonistic patterns that can occur when both contacts change simultaneously and to ensure the proper timing of the movement from distal to proximal.

Activity: Supine; unilateral D1F with knee flexing and D1E with knee extending

Technique: Slow reversal hold (SRH); MC thigh and foot

Impairments: Weakness of muscles in the D1 pattern; difficulty with control and reversing movements; abnormal movement in synergistic patterns.

114

Description

This is a mass pattern combining hip, knee, and ankle flexion with the reverse movement of hip, knee, and ankle extension. Movement of the *right* leg will be described. The patient is supine, positioned close to the edge of the plinth. The therapist stands near the patient's knee facing the head of the patient in the diagonal direction of the pattern. The therapist, with one MC on the heel and one under the thigh, guides the patient's limb through the pattern. D1F combines hip flexion, adduction, and external rotation, knee flexion, and foot dorsiflexion with inversion. The leg flexes in this mass pattern toward the opposite shoulder; the knee and foot cross the midline. D1E combines hip extension, abduction, internal rotation, knee extension, and foot plantarflexion with eversion.

To resist the pattern the limb is positioned in the lengthened range of the flexor pattern. The proximal contact is placed on the anterior medial thigh and the distal contact is on the anterior medial aspect of the foot with the therapist's fingers medial and the thumb lateral (Fig. 114A). All the components of the pattern are stretched and then resisted into the shortened range. In this range an isometric contraction is facilitated (Fig. 114B). While maintaining resistance with the proximal hand, the distal contact is pivoted to the plantar surface of the foot with the thumb under the toes. A stretch is applied to all the components of the extensor pattern, i.e., hip extensors, abductors, and internal rotators, knee extensors, foot plantarflexors, and ever-

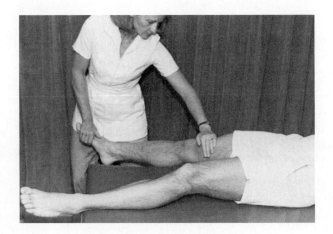

114A D1F knee flexion—lengthened range.

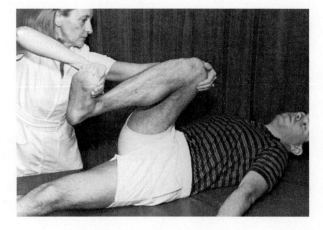

114B D1F knee flexion—shortened range.

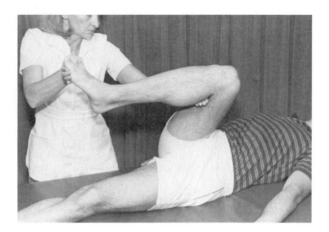

114C D1E knee extending—lengthened range.

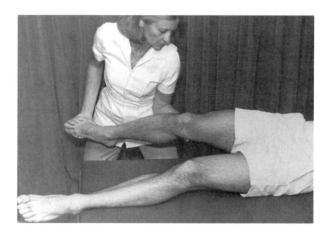

114D D1E knee extending—shortened range.

tors. Although the stretch is primarily provided by the distal hand, the proximal MC assists with the stretch by guiding the hip into more flexion and adduction. Following the stretch, as movement into the extensor pattern is initiated, the proximal, left, contact supinates, and the hand is placed on the posterior lateral thigh with the thumb lateral and the fingers medial (Fig. 114C). This proximal contact applies resistance with the web space of the thumb during the initial range of the extensor pattern, then with the palmar surface of the hand as the patient's leg fully extends. The hold applied in the shortened range of extension is enhanced by an approximation force (Fig. 114D). To reverse antagonists, the distal contact moves to the anterior surface of the foot. The pattern is stretched and movement initiated into the flexion range as the proximal contact then moves anteriorly and medially.

Purpose/Treatment Goals

The purposes are to facilitate a mass combination in the D1 pattern; to strengthen the iliopsoas, the hamstrings, and the anterior tibial muscles (D1F), the gluteus medius, the quadriceps, the gastrocnemius-soleus, and the peroneus longus (D1E); to promote a smooth reversal of antagonists and to enhance the skill level of control. The D1 pattern recombines the proximal components of the synergistic patterns.

Problems with Applications

Therapists frequently stretch only the distal component and not the entire pattern. The stretch to the extensor pattern should be toward the opposite shoulder incorporating stretch to the abductors as well as the extensors and rotators. The stretch to the flexor pattern incorporates traction and rotational elongation of the limb. In the shortened range of the flexor pattern knee flexion well beyond 90° is commonly allowed. At approximately 90 degrees of knee flexion adequate tension can be maintained in the hamstrings.

Activity: Supine; D1F, D1E knee straight
Technique: Slow reversal hold (SRH); MC thigh and foot
Impairments: Proximal muscles weakness; quadriceps weakness; difficulty combining dorsiflexion with knee extension; difficulty with reversing movements.

115

Description

In this activity the knee remains straight throughout the movement. The initial position of both the patient and the therapist is similar to that in the previous procedure. The patient's limb is moved through the flexor and extensor patterns with the knee remaining straight throughout the range. The range of the flexor pattern most likely will be limited by tightness of the hamstrings.

Straight leg pattern has a long lever arm increasing the challenge to proximal musculature.

   With MCs on the anterior medial thigh and foot, the movement is stretched and resisted in the lengthened range of the flexor pattern (Fig. 115A). The stretch, similar to the previous procedure, is a combination of traction, rotation, and movement into more hip and ankle extension. Because a long lever arm is created by the straight knee position, less resistance can be applied as compared with the mass flexor pattern. In the shortened range of flexion a holding contraction is resisted (Fig. 115B). To reverse the antagonists, the distal contact is moved first and the extensor pattern stretched and resisted. The proximal contact then moves to the posterior lateral surface of the thigh to provide resistance to the proximal muscles (Fig. 115C). Resistance should be provided equally with both the proximal and the distal contacts. In the shortened range of extension, the isometric contraction is enhanced by an approximation force (Fig. 115D).

Purpose/Treatment Goals

The purposes are to strengthen the hip muscles independently of the knee movement; to isometrically strengthen the quadriceps in their shortened range; and to promote dorsiflexion with the knee straight in preparation for the heel strike stage of the gait cycle.

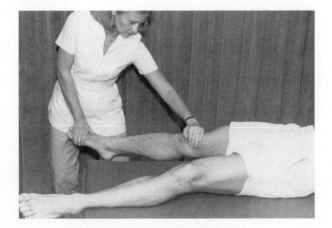

115A D1F knee straight—lengthened range.

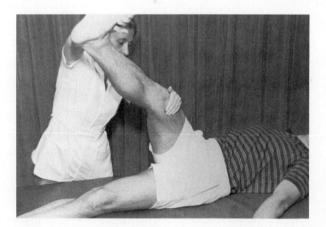

115B D1F knee straight—shortened range.

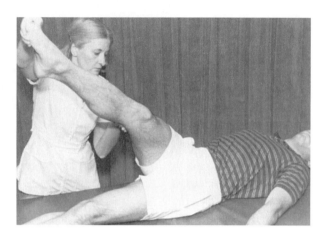

115C D1E knee straight—lengthened range.

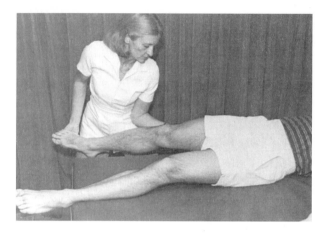

115D D1E knee straight—shortened range.

Problems with Application

If the patient has long legs, flexible hamstrings, or if the therapist is short, controlled movement toward the shortened range of the flexor pattern may be difficult. If such is the case the therapist should limit the range into flexion before control is lost. During the extension pattern resistance and support applied incorrectly with only the distal hand can force the knee into hyperextension.

116

Activity: Supine; unilateral D2F, with knee flexing, and knee straight
Technique: Slow reversal hold (SRH); MC thigh and foot
Impairments: Weakness of muscles in the D2 pattern; difficulty with reversing movements.

Description

The patient is positioned near the edge of the plinth with the limb in D2E, which combines hip extension, adduction, external rotation, and ankle plantarflexion and inversion. The other lower extremity should be abducted to allow adequate adduction of the exercising leg. The therapist is positioned at the patient's side facing the patient's foot in the diagonal direction of the pattern. The patient's leg is moved through the flexion pattern; the hip flexes, abducts, and internally rotates, the knee flexes and the ankle dorsiflexes and everts. The leg is returned to the extended position.

To stretch and resist the mass pattern, one MC is placed on the dorsal lateral aspect of the foot and the proximal MC is on the anterior lateral surface of the thigh (Fig. 116A). Because range into hip extension is limited by the plinth, the stretch is applied mostly to the rotational component at the hip and to the ankle movements. The limb is resisted into the shortened range of the mass D2F pattern where an isometric contraction is resisted (Fig. 116B). To reverse into the antagonistic extensor pattern, the distal MC is moved onto the plantar surface of the foot with the thumb under the toes and the extensor movement stretched. During the stretch the proximal contact must guide the thigh into more hip flexion and abduction while the distal contact stretches the foot and the knee. If the stretch is incorrectly applied to only the distal contact, a stress may be placed on the medial collateral ligament. Following the stretch, the therapist's proximal contact moves to the posterior thigh to resist the extensor pattern. This

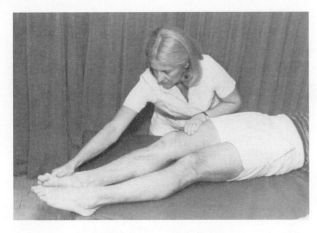

116A D2F—lengthened range.

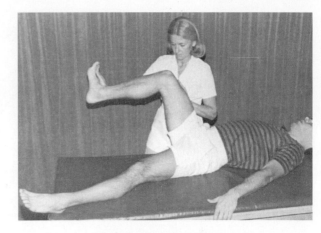

116B D2F—shortened range.

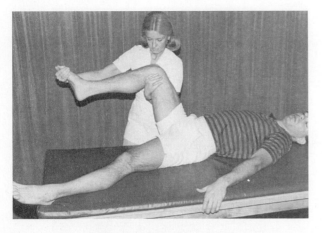

116C D2E—lengthened range.

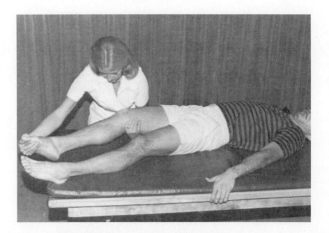

116D D2E—shortened range.

proximal contact approaches the thigh from the lateral side and should be positioned under, not over, the thigh (Fig. 116C). Approximation is applied in the shortened range of extension (Fig. 116D). To reverse the direction, the proximal contact maintains resistance to the extensor pattern as the distal contact is switched to the anterior surface of the foot to stretch the flexor movement and reverse the direction.

To perform the straight leg pattern, the contacts are in the same position but the knee remains straight throughout the pattern. The therapist may have to move with the patient's movement to allow full excursion of motion (Fig. 116E). The therapist may be positioned on the opposite side of the table to emphasize the lengthened range of the flexor pattern (Fig. 116F) or, more importantly, the shortened range of the extensor pattern (Fig. 116G).

Purpose/Treatment Goals

The purposes are to strengthen the tensor fascia latae, quadriceps, peroneus brevis (D2F); the gluteus maximus, hamstrings, gastrocnemius-soleus, and the posterior tibial (D2E); and to promote a smooth reversal of antagonists.

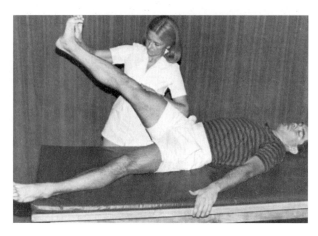

116E D2F—knee straight, shortened range.

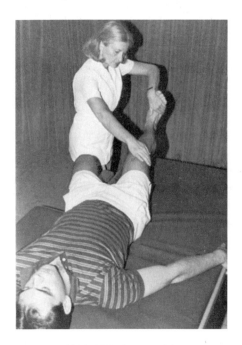

116F D2F—knee straight.

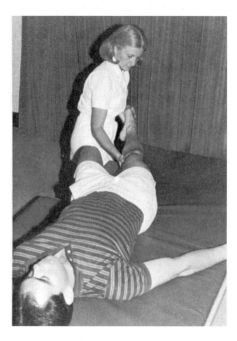

116G D2E—knee straight.

Problems with Application

Therapists may have problems with the placement of the distal MC during the flexion pattern. The forearm can be either supinated or pronated and the thumb medial or lateral, depending on which position is easier for the therapist.

The stretch in the lengthened range of the extensor pattern must be carefully applied so injury to the ligaments of the knee does not occur.

The proximal contact during the extension motion has to approach the thigh from the lateral aspect of the leg to ensure proper resistance throughout the range and to specifically resist *external* rotation with hip extension and adduction. This proximal contact may feel awkward in the beginning of the range but when the shortened range of extension is reached both MCs are resisting in the same direction and the movement can be more easily controlled.

Activity: Supine; D1F, knee flexing

Technique: Slow reversal hold (SRH) with timing for emphasis (TE), to hip and knee; MC thigh and foot

Impairments: Weak hip flexors or hamstrings.

Description

Specific techniques of emphasis can be applied to the unilateral patterns. TE is performed when an imbalance of strength exists in the pattern and the goal of the procedure is to strengthen the weakened musculature.

For the first example, TE is used if weakness of the hip flexors exists but the hamstrings and anterior tibial muscles are strong. The procedure begins either with resistance to the antagonist extensor pattern, which may facilitate the flexor pattern by successive induction, or with stretching in the lengthened range of the flexor pattern. This example will begin with stretch and resistance to flexion.

The leg is positioned in the lengthened range of D1 flexion and a stretch applied to all the components of the flexor pattern (Fig. 117A). The entire pattern is resisted but only the knee and the ankle flexor segments may be strong enough to achieve 90 degrees of flexion. In this range these stronger muscles are "locked in" with isometric resistance. Timing for emphasis is then performed to the hip flexors and adductors to facilitate their contraction through range (Fig. 117B). When the shortened range of hip flexion is achieved, an isometric contraction of the entire pattern is resisted and the reverse extensor motion is facilitated by stretch and resistance. In the shortened range of extension, the flexor pattern is again stretched and the sequence repeated. Because the hip flexors are moving against gravity, the therapist's resistance must be carefully applied if the muscles are below a 3/5 grade.

If the hamstrings are the weakest component of the flexor pattern, TE can focus on the knee flexors. The hip flexors, adductors, and dorsiflexor are resisted and "locked in" at 90 degrees, the range in which they can optimally hold. Timing for emphasis is applied to the hamstrings to improve knee flexion (Fig. 117C). During this flexor pattern the therapist's distal MC remains on the dorsum of the foot to sustain the isometric contraction of the ankle component. To resist the hamstrings with this distal MC the therapist lifts the foot up, attempting to extend the knee, and the patient responds by flexing the knee and pulling the foot down toward the op-

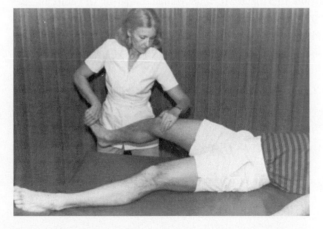

117A D1F—knee flexing—stretch lengthened range.

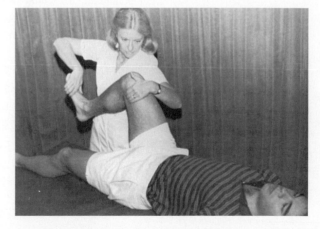

117B D1F—knee flexing—TE hip flexion, adduction.

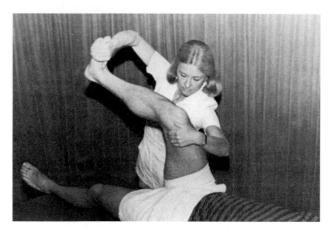

117C D1F—knee flexing; TE hamstrings.

posite knee. Because gravity is assisting knee flexion, this procedure is appropriate if the hamstrings are below 3/5. If the hamstrings are stronger, the prone patterns previously described are indicated.

Purpose/Treatment Goals

The purpose is to strengthen specific components of the pattern by maximizing overflow from the stronger muscles within the pattern. Mass movement combinations, hip, knee, and ankle flexion or extension, are most appropriate when strengthening is the goal of treatment as the intersegmental overflow seems to be greatest during these combinations.

Problems with Application

Therapists may not "lock in" the stronger components sufficiently prior to pivoting the weaker part. Overflow seems to be maximized when an isometric contraction of the stronger muscles is performed. The isometric portion of the technique, therefore, needs to be emphasized.

When the emphasis is on knee flexion the therapist may have difficulty with the distal MC and may incorrectly move the contact to the sole of the foot. To maintain resistance to the ankle component and to facilitate knee flexion, this distal MC must remain either on the anterior surface or the heel. If the contact is moved to the plantar surface of the foot, the extensor pattern rather than the flexor may be facilitated.

Activity: Supine; D1E, knee extending
Technique: Slow reversal hold (SRH) with timing for emphasis (TE), to hip and knee; MC thigh and foot
Impairments: Weak gluteus medius or quadriceps.

118

Description

In the D1E pattern emphasis can be directed to strengthening either the gluteus medius or the quadriceps muscles. To emphasize the hip component, the entire pattern is stretched and the strong knee and ankle extensors are resisted into their shortened ranges, where they are "locked in." This isometric contraction is facilitated by approximation. Emphasis then changes to the hip and all components of extension, abduction, and internal rotation are pivoted into the shortened range. (Fig. 118A). Because hip extension is assisted by gravity, manual resistance has to be sufficient to overcome the weight of the limb.

TE can be applied to knee extension when the quadriceps are the weakest component of the pattern. In this case the hip and the ankle are isometrically resisted in their shortened ranges and the quadriceps pivoted (Fig. 118B). Isometric resistance to "collapse" the entire leg into the flexor pattern is applied in conjunction with resistance to knee extension. The distal MC remains on the plantar surface of the foot with the therapist's thumb under the toes.

Purpose/Treatment Goals

The purpose is to strengthen the hip or knee extensors by maximizing overflow from stronger muscles within the pattern and emphasizing the weaker components.

TE also can be applied to the D2 pattern emphasizing either the flexion or extension direction if specific muscular weakness exists.

Problems with Application

The therapist may have difficulty maintaining the proper placement of the distal MC when emphasis is on the quadriceps. Overflow from the hip and the ankle extensors can occur only if this contact remains on the sole of the foot. If the distal contact is moved incorrectly to the anterior surface, the patient may tend to flex rather than extend the hip. If the quadriceps are above 3/5, a bilateral or unilateral pattern performed in sitting may be preferable.

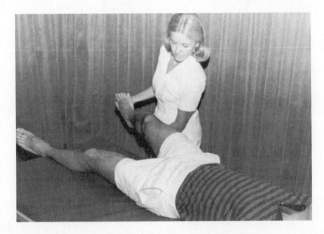

118A D1E—knee extending—shortened range.

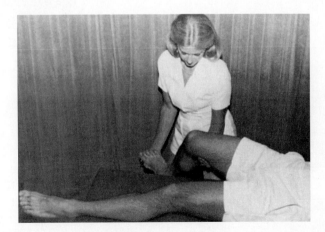

118B D1E—TE quadriceps.

119

Activity: Supine; D1E or D2E, knee straight
Technique: Slow reversal hold (SRH) with repeated contractions (RC); MC thigh and foot
Impairments: Weak gluteus medius or maximus.

Description

In either of the two diagonal patterns RC can be applied to strengthen the entire movement or to focus on the hip musculature. The procedure begins with stretch and resistance to the flexion pattern followed by stretch and resistance to the extensor pattern. Near the shortened range an isometric contraction is performed with approximation followed by RC of the entire pattern into more shortened ranges (Fig. 119A). With this activity the application of RC closely resembles that of TE. The goal is identical with both techniques, however, in this procedure all the movement components are repeated, no particular movement emphasized.

Purpose/Treatment Goals

The purposes are to strengthen the gluteus maximus (D2E) or the gluteus medius (D1E) with the knee straight and to strengthen all the muscles in the D1E or D2E patterns.

The technique of RC can be performed with an isometric contraction applied prior to the application of the repeated stretches. The purpose of the isometric contraction is to increase the stretch sensitivity of the muscles enabling them to respond more readily to the isotonic component of the technique.

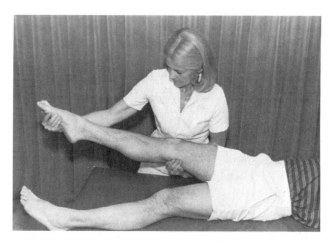

119A D2E—knee straight; RC.

Activity: Supine; D1 or D2 extension or flexion

Technique: Hold relax (HR); MC thigh and foot

Impairments: Decreased mobility of hip flexors or of hip extensors.

120

Description

HR can be applied to the two lower extremity patterns to increase the extensibility of the hip flexors. The technique can be applied with the patient in the Thomas test position or with the other LE in hooklying to stabilize the lower back and reduce the tendency to tilt the pelvis.

The leg is positioned in the lengthened range of hip flexion. With MCs on the posterior surface of the thigh and the foot, isometric resistance to the agonistic hip extensors is gradually increased, then released (Fig. 120A). Following relaxation, active range into more hip extension is resisted. The technique is repeated until no additional range into hip extension can be gained.

To increase range into hip flexion, the mass flexion pattern can be isometrically resisted followed by relaxation and active flexion motion.

Purpose/Treatment Goals

The purpose is to increase the extensibility of the hip flexors, specifically the iliopsoas in D1E and the tensor fascia latae in D2E, the hip extensors, and rotators. These muscles may need to be elongated in patients with low back dysfunction.

Problems with Application

When gaining range into extension the therapist may apply the isometric resistance to the antagonistic hip flexors. Although resistance to the antagonist may be appropriate in some procedures, in this activity, with the hip flexors on stretch, an isometric contraction of these muscles may result in an anterior tilt of the pelvis, an increased lumbar lordosis, or a strain at the sacroiliac joint. Weakness of the lower abdominals may exaggerate these unwanted movements. Even when the technique is properly applied to the agonist the lower back may need to be stabilized by the position of the other limb to avoid discomfort in this area.

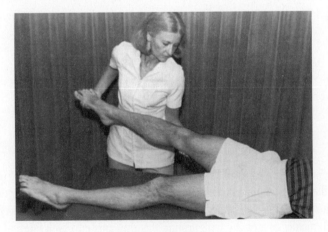

120A D1E; HR to agonist.

121

Activity: Supine; D1F or D2F knee straight

Technique: Hold relax (HR); MC thigh and foot

Impairments: Decreased mobility of hamstrings; limitations into SLR.

Description

HR can be applied to the D1 or D2F patterns to increase the extensibility of the hamstrings. The patient is positioned supine near the edge of the plinth. The limb is actively moved into either D1F or D2F. In the shortened range of the hip flexor pattern, an isometric contraction of the antagonistic hamstrings is resisted followed by relaxation and more movement into flexion. The technique is repeated until no additional range is gained. The therapist's MCs remain on the posterior surface of the limb during the isometric and relaxation portions of the technique and may be subsequently changed to the anterior surface to facilitate hip flexor motion. The therapist may stand on the opposite side of the plinth to better resist hamstrings in the shortened range of D1 flexion.

The agonistic hip flexors and knee extensors can be resisted to reciprocally inhibit the tight hamstrings. However, because of the long lever arm and the active insufficiency of the rectus femoris, more gains in range may be achieved with the hold applied directly to the antagonist.

HR is applied most commonly to a muscle in its lengthened range. However, gains in range can occur if the technique is applied in mid or even shortened ranges.

Purpose/Treatment Goals

The purposes are to increase extensibility of the hamstrings and range into SLR. Extensibility of this muscle group is needed if isolated tightness of the hamstrings decreases pelvic movement during functional activities and results in a focus of stress in the lower lumbar region. Superficial heating modalities and soft tissue techniques can be useful prior to the application of hold relax.

Problems with Application

The patient may attempt to push into extension rather than perform a graded isometric contraction. Micro tearing of the muscle may result from a sudden forceful increase in tension.

122

Activity: Supine; SLR or mass flexion motion

Technique: Rhythmical rotation (RR); MC thigh and heel

Impairments: Decreased mobility of hamstrings; tension of posterior structures.

Description

This passive technique can be used to gain ROM if the patient cannot actively participate in the exercise. With the patient supine on the plinth the therapist places MCs under the thigh and the heel. The leg is slightly raised off the mat so that the limb can be easily moved. The therapist slowly and rhythmically rotates the limb around the long axis into both internal and external rotation.

Purpose/Treatment Goals

The purpose is to maintain or gain range of motion in the hip and knee musculature.

This technique is most appropriate when the patient has difficulty actively contracting the involved musculature. Patients with complete SCI, Guillain–Barré syndrome (early stages), peripheral nerve injury, pain or extreme hypertonia may benefit from this technique.

Problems with Application

If the patient is incorrectly positioned, the low back of the therapist may be stressed. The patient should lie toward the edge of the plinth to improve body mechanics.

Activity: Supine; D1E, knee extending
Technique: Agonistic reversals (AR); MC thigh and foot
Impairments: Decreased eccentric control of quadriceps and hip extensors.

123

Description

The reversal of concentric and eccentric contractions of the prime movers in D1E can be facilitated with the technique of AR.

The procedure begins with the leg in the lengthened range of D1E. The hip and knee extensors are stretched and concentrically resisted into the shortened range, where a hold is applied. This is followed by resistance to an eccentric contraction of these same extensor muscles. The therapist's MCs remain on the posterior surface of the thigh and the plantar surface of the foot during the entire procedure. The verbal commands are "push down" (concentric contraction into the shortened range) (Fig. 123A), "hold" (isometric contraction in the shortened range of extension), "now make me work at bending your leg," or "slowly let your leg bend" (eccentric contraction from the shortened toward the lengthened ranges) (Figs. 123B, 123C). If the patient has difficulty controlling the lengthened range of the eccentric contraction, the technique is performed through increments of range, gradually increasing the range of the lengthening contraction.

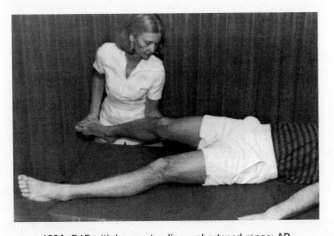

123A D1E with knee extending—shortened range; AR.

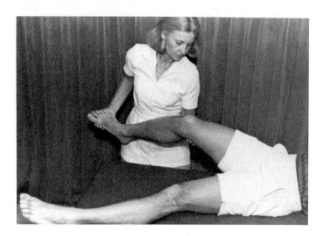

123B D1E—knee extending-mid range; AR.

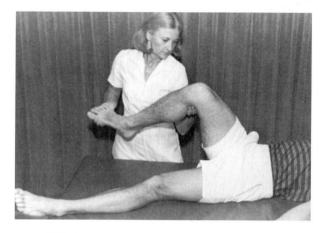

123C D1E—knee extending-lengthened range; AR.

Eccentric control of the quadriceps also can be promoted by AR to bilateral or unilateral movements in sitting.

Purpose/Treatment Goals

The purpose is to promote a smooth reversal of concentric–eccentric contractions of the extensors.

Eccentric control in the shortened ranges of knee extension is needed during ambulation. Activities, such as descending stairs or sitting from a standing position, require eccentric control in lengthened ranges of both the hip and knee extensors. Concentric–eccentric resistance can be provided primarily to the knee extensor portion of the pattern to isolate the quadriceps.

Problems with Application

Because reversal of antagonists has been previously emphasized, therapists may have difficulty maintaining MCs on one surface throughout the procedure.

124

Activity: Supine; D1F, knee flexing
Technique: Agonistic reversals (AR); MC thigh and foot
Impairments: Decreased eccentric control of hip and knee flexors.

Description

Concentric–eccentric control of the flexors may be facilitated using the mass flexion activity with the technique of AR. The therapist's MCs are positioned and maintained on the anterior thigh and the foot. The activity begins in the lengthened range of D1F where stretch and resistance to the flexion pattern is applied. As in the previous procedure an isometric contraction is resisted in the shortened range followed by an eccentric contraction of the same flexor muscle groups into lengthened ranges. The verbal commands are "bend your leg toward your opposite shoulder" (concentric), "hold" (isometric) (Fig. 124A), "now make it difficult for me to straighten your leg, or let your leg down slowly" (eccentric) (Fig. 124B). If the patient begins to

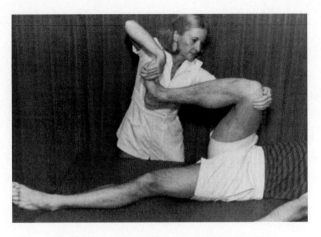

124A D1F with knee flexing—shortened range.

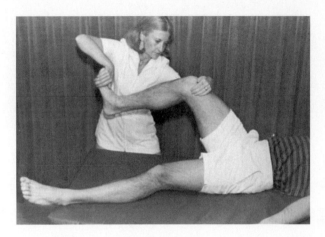

124B D1F—knee flexing-mid range; AR to flexors.

lose control in the lengthened range of flexion, the pattern is reversed back into the shortened range. The procedure is performed through increments of range as control is developed.

Purpose/Treatment Goals

The purpose is to facilitate eccentric control of the hip and knee flexors.

Eccentric control in the lengthened range of knee flexion is needed during the terminal swing phase of gait. AR, with emphasis in lengthened ranges of knee flexion, also can be promoted in sitting and may help to improve the stability provided by the posterior knee muscles in upright postures.

Activity: Supine; D1F with knee extending
Treatment: Slow reversal (SR); MC thigh and foot
Impairments: Abnormal timing of segments in an advanced combination.

125

Description

This procedure helps to promote the advanced combination of movement required during ambulation. It is incorporated into the treatment plan when the patient has sufficient strength to perform the movement but lacks coordination, timing, and proper sequencing of the components of the pattern.

The patient is positioned near the edge of the plinth with the lower leg flexed over the side. The therapist initially assists the patient through the pattern emphasizing the proper sequencing of the hip and knee components. Simultaneous hip flexion with knee extension and hip extension with knee flexion are desired. The therapist begins the procedure facing the patient's foot (Fig. 125A) then pivots with the limb movement (Fig. 125B). MCs are positioned on the anterior medial thigh and foot. The pattern is stretched and minimal resistance is applied to all components. When the shortened range is achieved, the distal contact is changed to the plantar surface of the foot to stretch the reverse movement; the proximal hand moves to the posterior lateral surface of the thigh and both contacts resist the movement (Figs. 125C, 125D). Because the proper sequencing of the movement combinations is difficult, many patients may need to be guided through the pattern.

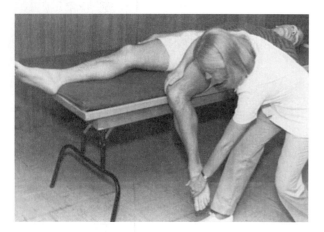

125A D1F with knee extending—lengthened range.

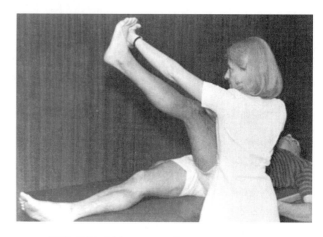

125B D1F with knee extending—shortened range.

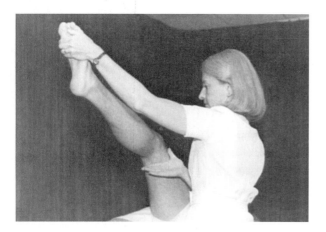

125C D1E with knee flexing—lengthened range.

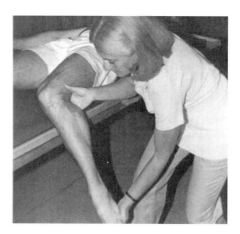

125D D1E with knee flexing—shortened range.

Purpose/Treatment Goals

The purpose is to promote the skill level of control by improving the timing and sequencing of movements within the pattern.

At this level of control, less sensory input should be needed to facilitate the activity. Tracking resistance is applied to guide the patient in the correct movement. If the patient does not have sufficient strength to perform this procedure, a less difficult procedure such as a mass pattern with the technique of TE, RC, or SRH is preferred. This advanced pattern is a total recombination of synergistic patterns.

Problems with Application

Instead of simultaneously performing the movements of the hip and knee joints, the patient may sequentially extend the knee then flex the hip resulting in a straight leg pattern. Similarly, during the reversal motion the patient may flex the knee after the hip is fully extended. To promote the desired coordinated response, the therapist should emphasize the verbal commands of "lift your thigh off the mat" during the flexion (hip) phase and "bend your knee" during the extension (hip) phase. The therapist may reinforce the patient's tendency to perform a modified straight leg pattern if too much resistance is applied.

The previous three procedures have been performed in the D1 pattern. It is possible, although difficult, to incorporate the techniques of AR with a mass D2 pattern and to perform the advanced combination in D2. Therapists may find it easier to learn these procedures in the D1 pattern.

The emphasis of the previous unilateral procedures has been on strengthening specific muscles, promoting concentric–eccentric control, and enhancing the timing or sequencing of the movement patterns. When developing and progressing a treatment plan, the therapist may choose these unilateral patterns to maximize overflow within the limb whereas the trunk and bilateral patterns can promote overflow from one limb to the other. All combinations can be incorporated into treatment or one combination may be most effective. Evaluating the patient's pattern of muscle strength and response to the procedures will indicate which activities are most beneficial.

The following procedures are designed to promote ankle and foot control. In these activities the proximal components are resisted to promote overflow into the weak distal segment. Initially the distal segment may be enhanced most effectively in a mass pattern. To progress, the distal movements are performed with varied proximal motions and in advanced patterns.

Activity: Supine; D1F with knee flexion

Technique: Timing for emphasis (TE) on ankle dorsiflexion with inversion; MC lower leg and foot

Impairments: Decreased concentric control of anterior tibialis.

126

Description

This procedure promotes strengthening of ankle dorsiflexion and inversion, primarily the tibialis anterior muscle. The patient is positioned in the middle of the plinth and the therapist stands near the foot of the plinth. The therapist's MCs are positioned on the posterior surface of the lower leg and on the anterior foot. All the components of the D1F pattern are stretched, with emphasis on the distal component (Fig. 126A). The leg is resisted into mass flexion and the heel placed on the plinth to provide the therapist better control of the ankle motion. In midrange the proximal hip and knee flexors are "locked in" by resistance provided by the MC on the calf. The distal contact on the foot then emphasizes concentric contractions to the ankle motion (TE) (Fig. 126B). After a few repetitions of movement into dorsiflexion and inversion, an

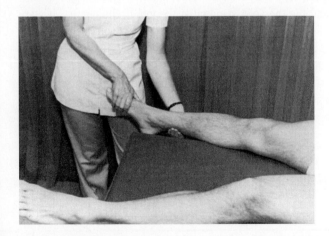

126A D1F—lengthened range; TE, ankle.

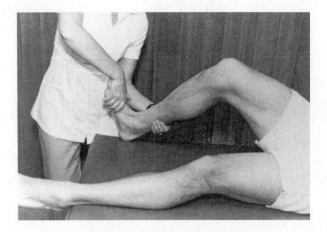

126B D1F—mid range; TE, ankle.

isometric contraction is performed to the entire pattern and the reversal motion of D1E stretched and resisted. The reversal movement is not emphasized.

The verbal commands are "bend your leg" (the therapist stretches and resists the pattern), "now keep it there" (the therapist locks in the proximal components, with the heel on the plinth), "now bend your ankle up and keep bending" (repeated contractions applied to the ankle muscles), "hold it" (as the shortened range is achieved in the ankle), and "now straighten your leg" (the pattern is reversed).

Purpose/Treatment Goals

The purpose is to strengthen the anterior tibialis and toe extensors in a mass flexion pattern.

For patients demonstrating synergistic influences in the lower extremity, the amount of flexion of the proximal components is gradually decreased until the patient can dorsiflex with the hip and knee near full extension. This recombination of patterns more closely simulates the movements needed during the heel strike phase of gait. This procedure also can be performed in a sitting position. In sitting the amount of proximal flexion can be gradually decreased by raising the height of the supporting surface or moving the patient closer to the edge of the chair extending the knee.

Dorsiflexion is promoted with the proximal components in progressively less flexion.

Problems with Application

With both MCs placed distally on the limb the reversal movement may be difficult to resist. Performing the reversal movement, however, may allow the flexor pattern to be more easily repeated through successive induction.

127

Activity: Supine; D2F with knee flexion
Technique: Timing for emphasis (TE) on ankle dorsiflexion with eversion; MC lower leg and foot
Impairments: Decreased concentric control of peroneus brevis.

Description

This procedure is similar to the previous one but differs in that the emphasis is now on the motion of dorsiflexion and eversion, specifically the peroneus brevis muscle. With the patient positioned in the center of the plinth and the therapist standing at the foot of the plinth, MCs are placed on the posterior surface of the lower leg and on the anterior lateral surface of the foot (Fig. 127A). All components of the D2F pattern are stretched and resisted until the heel is in contact with the plinth. The proximal components are then locked in and the distal component pivoted with repeated contractions (TE) (Fig. 127B). After a few repetitions of movement into dorsiflexion and eversion, an isometric contraction is performed to the entire pattern and the reversal movement is stretched and resisted.

Purpose/Treatment Goals

To strengthen the peroneal muscles, particularly the peroneus brevis. To make the procedure more difficult as with the preceding procedure, the pattern is repeated with less flexion of the proximal components until the ankle motion occurs with the knee straight.

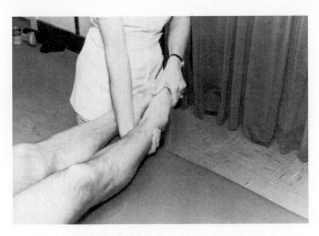

127A D2F—lengthened range; TE, ankle.

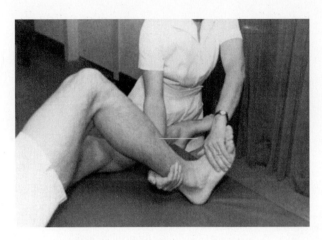

127B D2F—shortened range; TE, ankle.

Balanced dorsiflexion with both inversion and eversion is a goal for many patients with central nervous system deficits. Because inversion may be a part of the patient's abnormal movement, this D2F pattern, which emphasizes dorsiflexion with eversion, is an important part of advanced rehabilitation procedures. This movement of the limb is at the skill level of control. It is incorporated into the treatment plan when the emphasis is on timing and sequencing of the distal component that occurs during the swing and early stance phases of gait.

For patients who have experienced stress to the lateral structures of the ankle, strengthening into eversion is an important aspect of treatment.

In either of these two procedures the focus can be placed even more distally on the toe extensors. The proximal hand is positioned on the forefoot and the distal or pivoting hand is on the toes.

Although not described here, the distal components in the extensor patterns can be emphasized. The procedure is performed in a similar manner as that described for the flexor patterns. MCs are, as always, placed above and below the joint to be emphasized, the proximal components are locked in, and the muscles to be strengthened are stretched and resisted concentrically. The muscles primarily activated are the posterior tibial in D2E and the peroneus longus in D1E.

Problems with Application

The difficulty with the placement of MCs is the same as that discussed for the preceding procedure.

128

Activity: Supine; D1, D2F with knee flexion
Technique: Agonistic reversals (AR) to ankle; MC lower leg and ankle
Impairments: Inability to control eccentric contractions of dorsiflexors, invertors, evertors.

Description

This procedure promotes concentric–eccentric contractions of the distal components, the tibialis anterior in D1F and the peroneus brevis in D2F. As in the preceding procedures, MCs are on the lower leg and foot and the pattern is resisted to the point where the heel is on the plinth. At that point concentric–eccentric reversals of the ankle are resisted. The verbal commands may be "bend your leg and hold it" (lock in the proximal components), "pull up your ankle" (concentric ankle flexion), and "now make it difficult for me to pull it down or to straighten your foot" (eccentric ankle flexion). AR may be performed through increments of range.

Purpose/Treatment Goals

The purpose is to enhance concentric–eccentric reversals of the dorsiflexors in the D1F and D2F patterns. Eccentric control is primarily important for patients demonstrating a foot slap or a loss of control at the heel contact phase of gait. The extensor pattern can be used to promote eccentric control of the plantarflexors.

129

Activity: Supine; D1F knee extending
Technique: Normal timing (NT); MC thigh and foot
Impairments: Abnormal timing and sequencing of ankle movements with intermediate and proximal segments.

Description

This activity is similar to the advanced combination described earlier (Procedure 125), but in this procedure the technique is changed to emphasize the ankle movement. NT of movement proceeds in a distal to proximal progression, i.e., the distal component leads and the proximal components follow. Normal strength in all the muscles of the pattern as well as proper timing of proximal components has been achieved with previous procedures. The patient functionally may display a lack of proper sequencing or timing in the distal component, as evidenced by difficulty with the initiation of dorsiflexion during the beginning of the swing phase of gait.

To perform the procedure the patient is positioned near the side of the plinth and the lower leg is flexed over the edge. The therapist's MCs are on the anterior medial lower leg and the foot. The entire D1F pattern is stretched with emphasis on the distal component (Fig. 129A). The proximal movement is initiated but the therapist limits the amount of hip flexion and knee extension until the distal ankle component is activated and completes its range (Fig. 129B). The ankle movement is facilitated with verbal cues, quick stretches and minimal resistance. Once the distal segment responds the pattern is completed, facilitated by tracking resistance. During this movement the therapist maintains minimal resistance distally, otherwise the patient tends to "lose" the distal contraction.

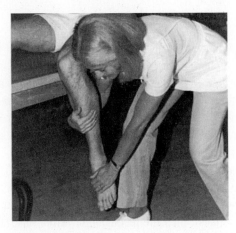

129A D1F, knee extending—lengthened range; NT.

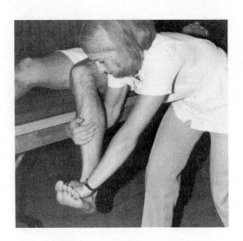

129B D1F, knee extending; NT.

Purpose/Treatment Goals

The purpose is to promote the normal distal to proximal timing of the movement in an advanced pattern.

This procedure may be difficult for the patient to perform because it combines dorsiflexion with knee extension. This functional combination is an advanced pattern rather than a mass pattern in which the distal component was previously strengthened (Procedure 126). Flexion of the hip, extension of the knee and ankle dorsiflexion should occur simultaneously and not sequentially. If this advanced pattern is too difficult, an intermediate step between mass flexion and this advanced movement can be added. The range of the proximal components during mass flexion gradually can be decreased until ankle dorsiflexion occurs with the hip and knee straight. Once this is performed, the advanced pattern just described can be attempted.

This is a skill level activity with a skill level technique, one of the most difficult procedures for the patient to perform. Therefore, tracking and guided resistance will be most appropriate to enhance the movement. At this advanced stage of treatment the goal is to withdraw the sensory input that at one time was necessary to facilitate the movement.

Problems with Application

Excessive resistance will reduce the patient's ability to perform the proper sequencing of this activity.

Summary

The procedures described in this text are those that, in the authors' experience, can be used to improve a wide variety of impairments. Once the reader develops skill applying the basic procedures and acquires a fundamental understanding of the techniques and their indications, other procedures can easily be formulated according to each patient's needs. The following are guidelines for choosing procedures to promote the different stages of control.

MOBILITY

Mobility includes both the ability to initiate movement and the presence of adequate ROM through which to move. To promote mobility, choose *activities*—postures, in which the BoS is large and the CoG is low. The movements performed in these postures may be total body activities, such as rolling or trunk, bilateral, or unilateral patterns. When the *initiation of movement* is desired, combinations that will maximize overflow may be appropriate, e.g., lower extremity, mass patterns can promote intersegmental overflow. To *increase ROM* activities are chosen that will maximize patient relaxation and the therapists' control of the involved segment.

Range of motion: The *techniques* of *hold relax, contract relax,* and *rhythmic stabilization* can be applied to any pattern or movement to increase ROM or extensibility of muscle tissue.

If ROM is limited and the patient does not have the ability to actively contract the musculature (as needed in the aforementioned techniques), then the technique of *rhythmical rotation* can be applied. In this technique the extremity is slowly and rhythmically rotated around the long axis of the limb for approximately 10 to 15 seconds. For example, to increase the range of SLR, the LE is passively rotated into internal and external rotation with the limb raised a few inches off the mat. The increase of range gained with this technique may be longer lasting than isolated passive stretch of the hamstrings.

Initiation of movement: For patients with increased tone or who have motor learning difficulties, the technique of *rhythmic initiation* is appropriate to initiate movement. This technique has been explained in conjunction with the total patterns of rolling and lower trunk rotation but can be used with all nonweight-bearing activities and all extremity patterns.

Hold relax active movement is used to initiate movement particularly of weak extensor muscles. The technique can be used in conjunction with rolling and LTR patterns and can be combined with other mat and extremity patterns. For example, it can be easily applied to the D1E pattern with knee extension to facilitate gluteus medius activity.

Repeated contractions is effective in initiating movement particularly of flexor muscles and can be used in conjunction with both mat and extremity patterns. This technique, which incorporates repeated stretches and resistance can be applied in the lengthened range of flexor patterns to initiate movement of weak muscle groups.

STABILITY

The stability stage of control is divided into two levels: muscle holding performed first in nonweight-bearing activities, and postural stability promoted in weight-bearing postures.

The *technique* of a *shortened held resisted contraction* can be applied to extensor patterns or individual muscles such as quadriceps or gluteals when muscle holding is the goal. SHRC is applied to one side of a joint. *Alternating isometrics* can be used when isometric strengthening around a joint is indicated. *Rhythmic stabilization* which incorporates isometric resistance to all components can, along with AI, improve stability in all weight-bearing postures.

CONTROLLED MOBILITY

Controlled mobility, the third stage of control, superimposes movement onto the stability developed in weight-bearing postures. During these weight-shifting motions, dynamic balance in the posture is promoted. Control of rotation within the segments of the trunk is also considered controlled mobility. The end goal of controlled mobility is the ability to assume various positions and to move within and between postures.

Slow reversal or *slow reversal hold* applied to weight-bearing activities promotes weight shifting, dynamic balance and, when performed through increments of range, the ability to independently assume the posture.

In weight-bearing activities *agonistic reversals* is most appropriately applied to improve the eccentric control of extensor muscles and to improve the ability to lower body weight within the posture.

SKILL

Skill implies manipulation of the environment with the upper extremities or locomotion with the lower extremities. Both of these functional activities require proper sequencing and timing of muscle activity. Speech is the skill level of oral motor function.

Appropriate *activities* are those in which the distal component is free to move, such as occurs with the extremity patterns. Skill can also be enhanced with ambulatory procedures.

The *techniques* include *resisted progression* which is applied to locomotive activities to improve ambulation control. *Normal timing* is used with individual patterns of movement to promote the distal to proximal sequencing of movement. *Slow reversal* or *slow reversal hold* enhances the smooth reversal of antagonistic muscle groups. Agonistic reversals combines concentric and eccentric contractions.

STRENGTHENING

Strength is an integral part of each stage of control. Strengthening can include improved neural transmission, muscular coordination, learning or actual hypertrophy of muscle tissue. The techniques of *slow reversal hold, timing for emphasis,* and *repeated contractions* combine repetition, overflow, and resistance, all of which can affect the strength of the response. These techniques are most commonly applied to trunk, bilateral, or unilateral extremity patterns but are also appropriately applied to certain mat activities such as, upper or lower trunk movements.

Study Questions

Match the impairments with the appropriate treatment procedure. More than one procedure may be appropriate for an impairment.

Impairments	Procedures
1. Ankle stability (initial stage)	Activity: Sitting; LE, D2F unilateral Technique: AI RS
2. Decreased ROM into elbow extension	Activity: Supine; UE, D1E Technique: HR
3. Positive Trendelenburg gait	Activity: Bridging Technique: AI RS
4. Weak wrist and finger extensors	Activity: Supine; UE D1 thrust Technique: TE
5. Weakness in opponens pollicis	Activity: Supine; UE D2E Technique: TE
6. Decreased ROM into hip extension	Activity: Sidelying; LE D1E Technique: HR

Impairments	Procedures
7. Decreased stability of low back extensors	Activity: Quadruped; LE D1E Technique: SRH emphasis shortened range
8. Decreased ROM into shoulder flexion and abduction	Activity: Sitting: UE D2F Technique: HR
9. Decreased eccentric control of hip extensors	Activity: Bridging Technique: AR

Worksheets

CASE #1

Mrs. J is a 65-year-old woman who fell on the ice and fractured her dominant right proximal humerus one week ago. She had just retired from a secretarial job. She lives at home with her husband, and two grown children. She is slightly hypertensive which is medically controlled. She is anxious to begin therapy and regain functional use of her arm. She states she is afraid of walking outside since her fall.

Her pain is minimal to moderate with attempts to move her arm and she cannot sleep on the right side. She is in a sling that can be removed only for her exercise sessions. The relevant findings from examination of her physical systems include:

ANS—slight anxiety, no sign of cold or sweaty palms
CVP—slight hypertension
MS-ROM—active assisted-flexion 60, abduction 30, internal rotation full, external rotation –10. All muscles intact
Movement control—excessive scapular elevation and abduction upon attempts to lift arm
Movement capacity—previous walking distance about 1 mile
Sensation—intact and equal bilaterally

Your impression from the initial evaluation is that she is generally in good health and because of her excellent cognition, motivation, and family support she will comply with a home exercise program. You decide to have her continue her exercise program at home until bone healing allows more active therapy.

Her initial home exercise program will focus on increasing or maintaining control in areas proximal and distal to the involved segment, and maintaining or improving specific muscle endurance and general body capacity.

To improve or maintain scapular control you consider the motions most commonly problematic. Scapular elevation and abduction are excessive during arm elevation. To discourage this tendency what motions need to be emphasized?_____. Because these movements provide scapular stability, isometric contractions in shortened ranges are emphasized even during this early phase of rehabilitation. To avoid stress on the humerus, isometric contractions initially are performed without external resistance. To improve muscle stability how long should the patient hold the contraction?_____. Why?_____. How much effort, percent of a maximum contraction, would you have the patient perform?_____. Why? _____. In what posture (s), supine, sitting, or standing would you have the patient perform these scapular motions?_____. Why?_____ (Procedures_____, Fig._____).

You encourage the patient to move the gleno-humeral joint by active assisted movement.

Assistance can be provided by gravity with Codman's exercises and by the uninvolved limb with an assisted D1 thrust. During this motion she is encouraged not to excessively elevate her scapula. Why do you have her assisting with her uninvolved limb?_____(Procedures_____, Fig._____). Distal movements of the elbow wrist and hand are performed actively.

A general walking program is encouraged to improve general body capacity. Because she is anxious about falling she is encouraged to walk with her husband or a friend until her comfort level improves. If cold weather is a problem, walking inside at a gym, mall, or other protected environment is suggested.

She returns four weeks postfracture with an x-ray report of good callus formation indicating that therapy can be more aggresive. She has been performing her home exercises twice a day and walking indoors about 30 minutes, 4 times a week. You determine that she should come for therapy twice a week for the next few weeks.

Her ROM and strength assessments are: Flexion 80 degrees, abduction 60 degrees, internal rotation full, external rotation 5 degrees. Because the bone is not fully healed strength assessment is performed by observation or assisted active movement. You assess that she has approximately 3/5 strength of all shoulder motions. Scapula strength, with resistance provided proximally, is approximately 4/5. Distally the resistance also is modified and a strength assessment of 4/5 is determined. During the active movements, excessive scapular elevation is still noted.

Her *functional limitations* are reported to be difficulty with dressing particularly putting on sweaters, coats, bra; she cannot reach beyond the first shelf of her cupboard, and she cannot perform household ADL or drive her shift car. *Treatment goals* include: increasing ROM, strength and stability around the scapulo-thoracic and gleno-humeral joints, and improving proximal dynamic stability (scapulo-humeral rhythm) and muscle endurance.

To increase her ROM you first want to continue the movements she has been performing at home. The *activity* is an assisted D1 thrust and performed in supine or sitting. What would be the advantages and disadvantages of each posture?_____. To increase range of tight muscles the *technique* of choice is_____. This can be performed to the agonist or the antagonist. Which would be most advantageous?_____. To increase range into the D1F which muscles are the agonist?_____. Considering that bone healing is not complete and the need to avoid pain and muscle splinting, what should be the intensity of the contraction?_____ (Procedures_____, Fig._____). What technique may be used to increase extensibility of the capsule?_____. With what intensity would it be applied?_____. Which soft tissue technique could be used to increase superficial circulation and decrease tissue stiffness?_____. What thermal modalities might be used prior to or in conjunction with this procedure to increase tissue extensibility?_____.

The next treatment goal is to improve the muscle strength and stability around the glenohumeral and scapulo-thoracic joints. This may be initiated by improving the scapular and shoulder muscle stability. The first level of stability is_____. The technique to promote this ability is_____. The intensity of effort should be limited to about 40% of a maximum contraction. In what postures could this level of stability be performed by the patient as part of her home program. List these procedures_____ (Procedures_____, Fig._____).

To progress to postural stability what techniques can be performed?_____. These can be applied to the scapula and to the arm first in non-weight bearing then in weight bearing postures. What is a sequence of weight bearing postures in which the range at the shoulder and the amount of weight bearing is gradually increased?_____, _____, _____. (Procedures_____).

When healing is sufficient, controlled mobility and static-dynamic stages of control can be emphasized in these weight bearing postures. What is a sequence of techniques that would achieve the progressively more difficult stages of control?_____ Delineate the activities, postures and movements, and the techniques to achieve the controlled mobility and static-dynamic stages. (Procedures_____)

Describe how these procedures can be performed independently in the clinic and then incorporated into the home program._____

If you find specific muscle weakness, particular movements can be performed with strengthening techniques. Match the muscle to the pattern in which it is most active.

A   Serratus anterior   _____D1F
B   Middle trapezius   _____D1E
C   Middle deltoid   _____D2F
D   External rotators   _____D2E
E   Internal rotators

What are the indications for choosing a trunk, bilateral, or a unilateral movement?_____

Which techniques are specifically used to increase strength?_____

CASE #2

A patient you are treating has poor proximal stability both of the upper and lower trunk. This may be due to central nervous system involvement, disuse atrophy, or pain in the thoracic or lumbar regions. Although each of these will have particular concerns that need to be considered some generalizations can be made regarding the choice of procedures.

Muscle stability is best achieved by promoting isometric contractions in the shortened ranges of the one-joint postural extensor. The technique to promote muscle stability is_____. Describe the intensity and duration of the contraction when the goal is improved muscle stability.

This stability technique can be performed in a variety of non-weight-bearing postures. If the patient is weak, has pain, or if increased effort results in sustained abnormal responses, the posture chosen should minimize the challenge. The postures that provide the largest BoS and lowest CoG are_____, _____, _____. For different types of patients what are the advantages and disadvantages of each of these postures?_____.

What might you observe if the patient had difficulty with postural stability in sitting or standing?_____

To improve *postural stability* particularly in the lower body, which more advanced, weight-bearing postures could be incorporated into treatment?_____. To promote upper body stability what additional postures could be used?_____ What techniques promote postural stability?_____. What are the biomechanical and neurophysiological factors that vary with these progressive postures?_____.

CASE #3

Your patient is a 30-year-old construction worker who suffered a stretch injury to his left axillary nerve three weeks ago when a 50-pound plank was dropped onto his shoulder. His sensation is normal and pain is minimal; the strength of the involved muscle(s) is 2/5.

• List the involved muscles
• For each muscle list the pattern in which it is optimally active
• List strengthening procedures for each of the involved muscles including the postures, movement patterns and combinations, and the techniques. Defend your choice of procedures.

CASE #4

Your patient is a 45-year-old nurse who fell and fractured her left proximal tibia 12 weeks ago. She is out of her cast and weight bearing to tolerance with crutches. Her impairments include decreased active and passive knee ROM (flexion 90 degrees, extension –10 degrees) with moderate pain at end ranges, and weakness of hip, ankle (4/5), and knee musculature (3–/5).

- In which postures can techniques to promote mobility best be performed?
- What are the advantages and disadvantages of each posture?
- What would be a sequence of mobility techniques?
- What is the rationale for their use?
- What would be a sequence of procedures to increase quadriceps and hamstring stability?
- What procedures could be used to specifically strengthen the quadriceps and hamstrings?
- Describe the procedures that could be performed as part of a home program to achieve the goals of improving ROM, increasing muscular stability around the knee, and strengthening the quadriceps and hamstrings.

CASE # 5, 6

You are treating two patients, one with quadriceps weakness following a total knee replacement and another with increased muscle tone and weakness of the quadriceps following a cerebral vascular accident. Describe the similarities and differences in the treatment of these two patients, including discussion of the following:

- Reflexes and their influence on your choice of postures.
- Inhibitory influences on the quadriceps; procedures to minimize or maximize their effects.
- Sensory inputs to enhance or to dampen the muscle's response.

Both these patients may have impaired mobility. Which aspects of mobility would most likely be affected with each?

Which techniques would be most appropriate for each mobility impairment?

Describe two ways to apply HR. What is the rationale for each of these applications?

Why might CR be inappropriate for patients with central nervous system dysfunction?

Why might muscle stability be impaired with each of these patients?

Which procedures could be used to improve muscle stability.

How might you modify the muscle stability technique for patients with CNS dysfunction?

Which techniques and weight-bearing postures would be appropriate to improve postural stability?

Which postures would you include for a sedentary 70-year-old person and which might you choose for an active 60-year-old person with the same problem?

Treatment
equipment

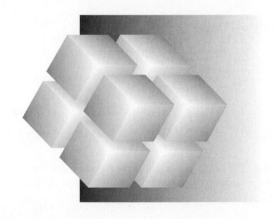

part
three

Equipment—Pulleys

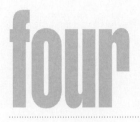

Chapter Outline

Introduction
Upper Body Movements
Lower Body Movements

Key Terms

Range of resistance
Direction of resistance
Traction
Compression

INTRODUCTION

Various types of equipment can be used as adjuncts to therapeutic procedures to augment the goals of treatment. A pulley system, common to most physical therapy departments is very versatile and can be modified to complement many therapeutic procedures. A resistive band can be substituted for pulleys and is an effective and practical way to exercise at home. Two factors must be controlled with pulleys: the range in which maximum resistance occurs and the direction of the resistive force.

To use pulleys effectively the therapist first must determine the range in which the maximum resistance is to be applied. Maximum resistance occurs at the point that the pulley line is at a 90-degree angle with the limb. When the angle is more acute, compression is combined with resistance; when the angle is more obtuse, traction with resistance occurs. Most pulley systems are arranged at different levels, for example, floor, shoulder, or overhead which allows for a variation in the angle of resistance. An elastic band also can be used at varying heights. Changing the patient's position relative to the pulley or elastic band also alters the angle of resistance.

Resistance can be applied to movement in a diagonal direction or altered to emphasize one plane of motion. The direction of resistance can be determined by observing the relationship of the pulley line to the limb in the beginning, middle, or end of the range. The pulley line may be aligned as direct extension of the limb (Figs. I-A, I-B) directly opposite the limb or directly overlying the limb.

For example, to perform straight flexion or extension movements the patient is positioned directly in front of the pulley. To resist diagonal movement the patient is angled diagonally in relation to the pulleys.

A reversal of concentric–eccentric contractions or AR is the technique primarily performed when moving against the resistance of the pulley system. In some situations a reversal of antagonists can also be added to the reversal of agonists. Examples will be noted throughout this section.

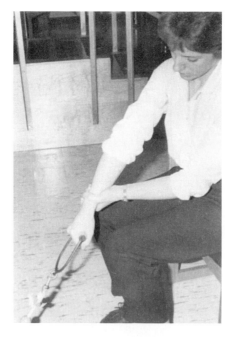

IA Floor level pulley.

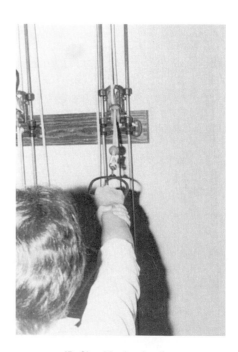

IB Shoulder level pulley.

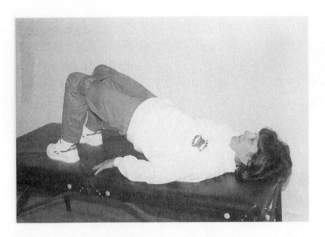

IC Bridging hip abduction, isometric contraction of one limb.

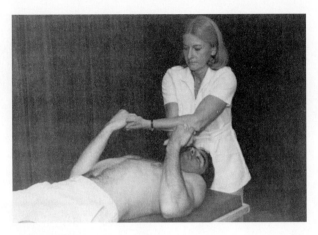

ID Increasing isometric resistance by moving further from the point of resistance.

Isometric contractions can be performed with both the resistive elastic band and pulley systems. Patients who are too weak to concentrically move against a force may be able to eccentrically contract or isometrically maintain a fixed position while band tension resistance is increased. Isometric resistance can be applied when the band is held taut between two limbs; one limb can perform concentric–eccentric movement while the other isometrically maintains a constant position. External rotation of the upper extremity and hip abduction are examples of these applications (Fig. I-C). The band also can be fixed to a door knob or some other stationary object while the patient isometrically maintains a limb position, for example, holding the scapula in adduction, while stepping away from the resistive force (Fig. I-D).

The following examples of pulley procedures illustrate how resistance and alignment can be effectively varied to successfully augment goals of treatment.

Upper Body Movements

Activity: Sitting; upper trunk extension (lift), facing the pulley
Technique: Agonistic reversals; floor level pulley

130

Description

In this procedure the patient is angled so that the pulley line is a direct extension of the leading D2 limb at the beginning of the range (Fig. 130A). Resistance is applied in a diagonal direction. At the beginning of the movement a traction force is applied. As the lift is performed, maximum resistance occurs when the UEs approximate 90 degrees of flexion (Fig. 130B). In the shortened range of the lift, a compression force is combined with the resistance (Fig. 130C). This procedure can be resisted by elastic band (Fig. 130D).

Purpose/Treatment Goals

Strengthen upper back extensors, trapezius, middle deltoid, promote crossing of the midline, promote dynamic postural control, and weight shifting in sitting.

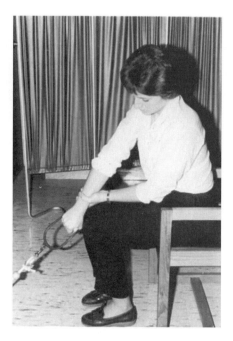

130A Lengthened range, a traction force.

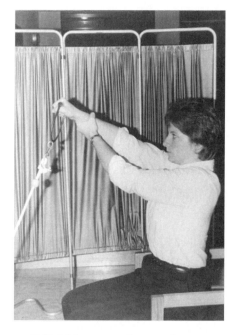

130B Midrange, maximum resistance.

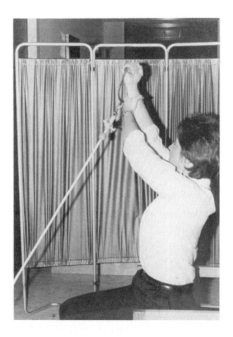

130C Shortened range, resistance with a compression force.

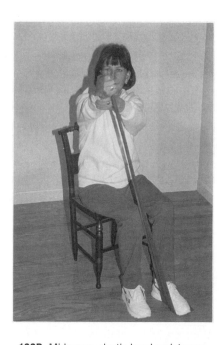

130D Midrange, elastic band resistance.

Activity: Sitting; upper trunk extension, lift, facing the pulley
Technique: Agonistic reversals, shoulder level pulleys

131

Description

The patient is at an angle to the pulley, as in the previous procedure. At the beginning of the range (90 degrees of shoulder flexion), a traction force occurs (Fig. 131A). Maximum resistance is applied in the shortened range of the lift (Figs. 131B, 131C). The direction of resistance is the same as in the previous procedure.

Whenever a traction force is applied in the midrange of the pattern, movement can occur in either direction from the midposition against resistance. In this example, movement can be resisted into the lift (shoulder flexion) or into the reverse lift (shoulder extension). If both directions from this midrange are performed the patient will be reversing antagonists. If the therapist's goal is to strengthen only one group of muscles, concentrically and eccentrically, then movement only in one direction is performed.

Purpose/Treatment Goals

Strengthen upper back extensors, lower trapezius, middle deltoid, and external rotators in shortened ranges; promote postural control in sitting.

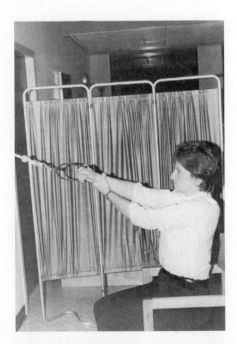

131A A traction force as the limb begins movement from midrange.

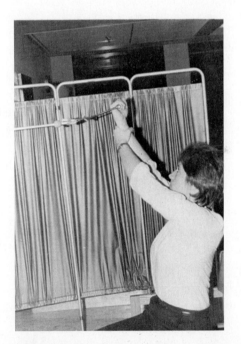

131B Maximal resistance provided in the shortened range.

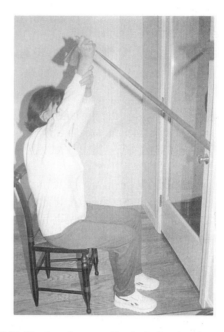

131C Shortened range with elastic band resistance.

132

Activity: Supine; upper trunk extension, lift, plinth parallel to the wall
Technique: Agonistic reversal

Description

The patient is supine on a plinth, positioned parallel to the wall. The range in which maximum resistance occurs can be altered by moving the plinth in relation to the overhead pulley. If maximum resistance in the shortened range of the lift is desired the plinth is positioned so that the pulley is directly above the hand when the limb is contracting in the shortened range (Figs. 132A, 132B). If a compression or approximation force is to be incorporated in the shortened

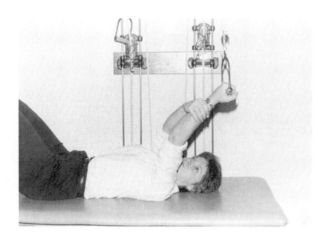

132A Beginning trunk extension movement.

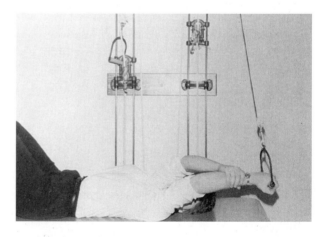

132B Maximum resistance provided in shortened range.

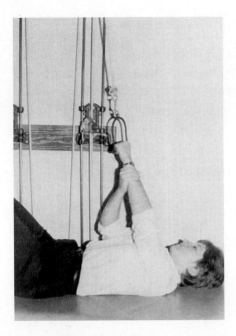

132C Beginning movement.

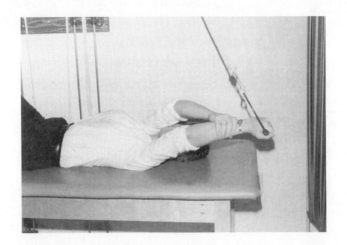

132D Compression force with resistance in shortened range.

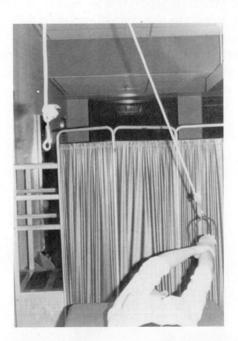

132E Angle of force increasing resistance to shoulder abduction.

range of the lift, the plinth is moved so that the pulley is aligned with the limb as the movement is initiated (Fig. 132C). An acute angle of resistance then occurs in the shortened range (Fig. 132D). Generally when maximum resistance is desired in one portion of the range, resisted movement through full range is sacrificed.

To resist the abduction component of the lifting pattern, the plinth is moved out from the wall to position the pulley line at about 45 degrees from vertical (Fig. 132E). With the plinth closer to the wall and the arms directly under the pulley, resistance is applied primarily to straight plane flexion.

A combination of two levels of pulleys (overhead and shoulder) can be used. The plinth remains parallel to the wall. Because of the angle of resistance the overhead pulley will primarily resist flexion and the shoulder level pulley will resist abduction. The result of the two resistive forces is a combination of the two directions of resistance.

Purpose/Treatment Goals

Strengthen upper trunk extensors and shoulder flexors in shortened ranges.

133

Activity: Sitting; upper trunk flexion with rotation (chop) diagonally facing the pulley

Technique: Agonistic reversals, shoulder level pulleys

Description

The patient is sitting diagonally facing the shoulder level pulleys. To resist the diagonal direction of the pattern the patient is at an angle to the pulleys. This can be accomplished in two ways. The chair can be placed directly in front of the pulleys and turned to a 45-degree angle or the chair can be placed parallel to the wall but moved to the side a few feet.

The height of the pulley determines where in the range maximum resistance occurs and, to some extent, the direction of the resistance. The shoulder level pulley is used so the pulley line is a direct extension of the limb, producing a traction force in the beginning of the range (Fig. 133A). In the midrange, maximum resistance occurs and compression is combined with resistance in the shortened range (Figs. 133B, 133C).

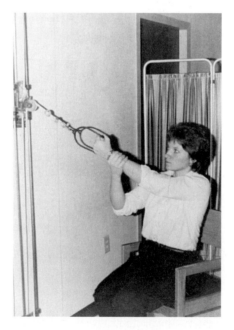

133A Range of initiation, traction force applied to the limb.

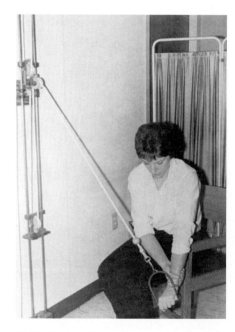

133B Shortened range, compression force combined with the resistance.

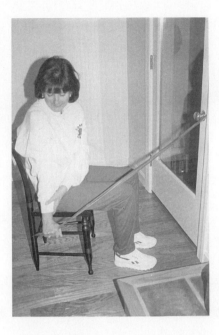

133C Shortened range with elastic band.

Purpose/Treatment Goals

Strengthen upper abdominals and shoulder extensors; promote crossing of the midline, weight shifting, dynamic postural control in sitting

Activity: Sitting; reverse of the trunk flexion pattern (reverse chop)
Technique: Agonistic reversals

134

Description

The patient is seated facing the pulleys. The chair can be positioned as in the previous procedure. The reverse chop can be resisted using the floor level pulleys. In the beginning of the range the pulley line is a direct extension of the limb (Fig. 134A). Maximum resistance occurs in midrange and some compression occurs in the shortened range (Fig. 134B).

When performing any of the trunk patterns in sitting, the patient's balance is challenged. If muscle strengthening is the primary goal then a more stable position, such as supine, may be more appropriate. However, sitting is the posture of choice to combine the goals of improved sitting balance, weight shifting and strengthening of the trunk and extremities.

Purpose/Treatment Goals

Strengthen upper trunk extensors, shoulder flexion with adduction; promote crossing of the midline, promote dynamic postural control and weight shifting in sitting.

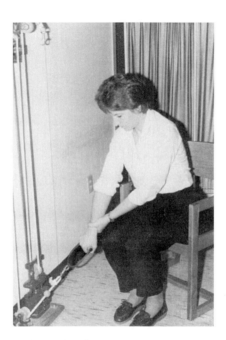

134A Traction force at the range of initiation.

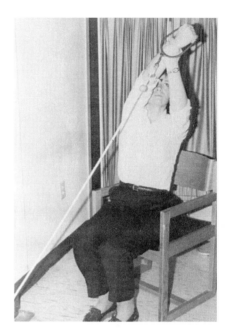

134B Compression force in the shortened range.

135

Activity: Supine; trunk flexion with rotation

Technique: Agonistic reversals, shoulder and overhead pulley

Description

In this procedure the patient is supine on the plinth with the plinth turned so that the patient's head is near the pulleys. The plinth is positioned in front of the pulleys at a slight angle to the wall or a few feet lateral to the pulley. The shoulder level pulley is used to provide traction in the lengthened range (Fig. 135A), maximum resistance in midrange, and compression in the shortened range (Fig. 135B). To increase the resistance to shoulder and elbow extension in the shortened range, the overhead pulley can be substituted (Fig. 135C).

The diagonal direction of resistance facilitates the oblique abdominal muscles. This is particularly effective for patients with paraparesis as it incorporates the functional goal of improved rolling with a treatment goal of strengthening the abdominals. To accentuate the rotational component of rolling, the plinth is turned more parallel to the wall (Fig. 135D). In this position the arms move into more abduction–adduction and the resistance to upper trunk rotation is increased (Fig. 135E).

Purpose/Treatment Goals

Strengthen upper abdominals and shoulder extensors, promote overflow from stronger upper limbs to weaker abdominals.

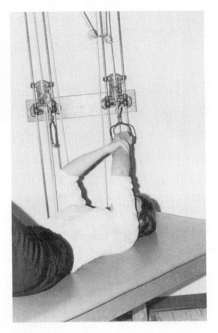

135A Traction force at the range of initiation.

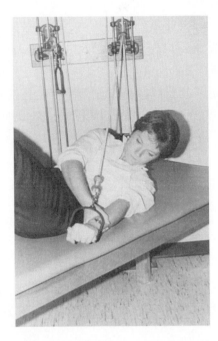

135B Compression force in the shortened range; the resistive force is focused on the abdominals not the leading limb.

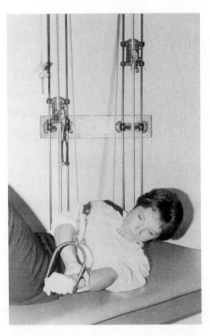

135C Overhead pulley decreasing compressive force and increasing resistance to shoulder extension.

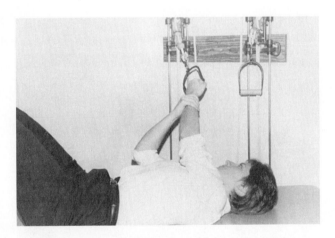

135D Direction altered to increase resistance to rotation.

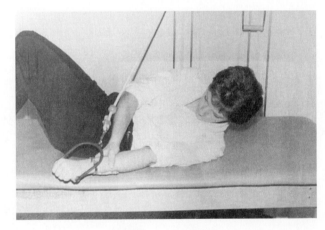

135E Shortened range.

136

Activity: Sitting; bilateral symmetrical D2F, facing the pulley
Technique: Agonistic reversals, floor and shoulder level pulleys

Description

To increase the difficulty of the procedures, the sequence of limb patterns usually progresses from trunk, to bilateral, to unilateral combinations. The bilateral pattern of BS D2F would therefore follow the lifting movement in a treatment program.

The patient is sitting directly in front of the pulleys holding onto the opposite pulley handles. Either the floor or shoulder level pulleys can be used. With the floor level pulleys, traction occurs at the beginning of the movement (Fig. 136A), maximum resistance occurs in midrange (Fig. 136B), and compression is combined with resistance in the shortened range (Fig. 136C).

With the shoulder level pulleys, the point of maximum resistance changes. Traction occurs in midrange (Fig. 136D) and maximum resistance occurs in the shortened range of the D2F pattern (Fig. 136E). From the midrange D2F also can be resisted with an elastic band (Fig. 136F).

Holding onto the opposite pulley lines is necessary to resist the diagonal direction of movement. If the pulley directly in front of the limb is used, resistance is provided primarily to shoulder flexion.

Purpose/Treatment Goals

Strengthen trapezius, middle deltoid, external rotators in mid- to shortened ranges, promote trunk extension.

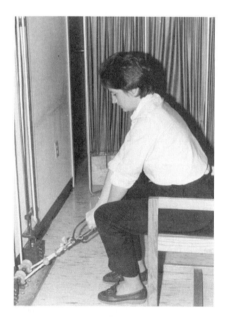

136A Traction force in the range of initiation.

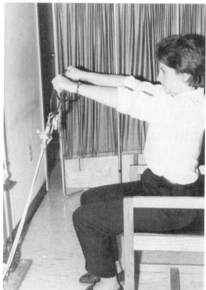

136B Maximum resistance in midrange provided by the floor level pulleys.

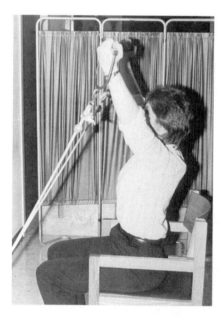

136C Compression force combined with resistance in the shortened range.

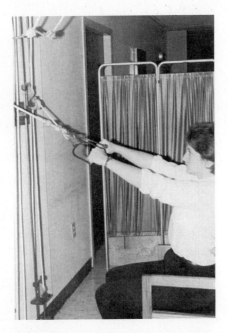

136D Shoulder level pulleys provide a traction force in midrange.

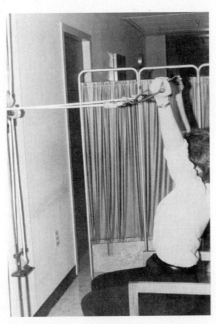

136E Maximum resistance provided in shortened range by the shoulder level pulleys.

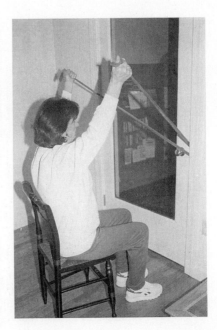

136F Resisting shortened range with elastic band.

Activity: Sitting or standing; bilateral symmetrical D1E and D1 withdrawal, facing the pulleys

Technique: Agonistic reversals

137

Description

The shoulder level pulleys provide maximal resistance to shoulder and elbow extension in the shortened range of D1E (Figs. 137A, 137B). The overhead pulleys produce a compression force through the arm and maximally resist scapula depression in the shortened range (Fig. 137C). To resist the diagonal direction of the pattern the opposite pulley lines are used. Elastic band resistance can resist these bilateral combinations (Fig. 137D).

Purpose/Treatment Goals

Strengthen thoracic extensors, scapular adductors, shoulder and elbow extensors, promote sitting or standing dynamic postural control. In sitting endurance or strengthening can be promoted by either increasing the number of repetitions of the procedures or the amount of weight; in standing postural control can be challenged as the changing CoG is maintained within the BoS.

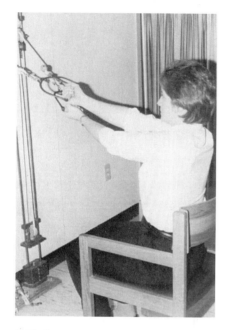

137A Sitting shoulder level pulleys, lengthened range.

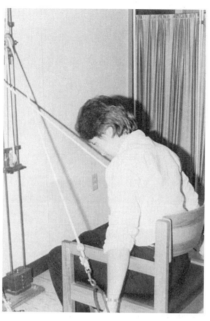

137B Shortened range of extensor pattern.

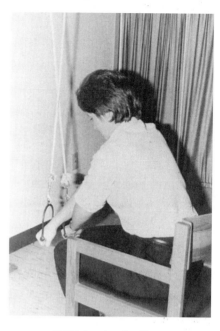

137C Overhead pulleys.

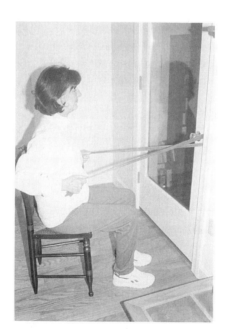

137D Sitting with band resistance, shortened range.

Activity: Sitting; unilateral upper extremity patterns
Technique: Agonistic reversals

138

Description

As with the trunk and bilateral patterns, all unilateral patterns can be resisted by using the three different levels of pulleys. To resist extensor motions either the overhead or the shoulder level pulley is used. The overhead pulley resists scapula depression and the shoulder level pulley resists primarily the shoulder extension component in the shortened ranges (Figs. 138A, 138B). To resist shoulder flexion patterns the floor level pulleys are used when maximum resistance is desired in midrange. In lengthened and shortened ranges traction and compression forces are added to the resistance (Figs. 138C, 138D). Theraband resistance can be used to resist shoulder flexion in mid range (Fig. 138E).

Purpose/Treatment Goals

Improve endurance and strenthen upper trunk and upper extremity musculature, promote sitting postural control.

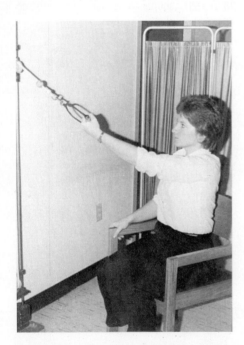

138A D1E lengthened range, traction force provided by shoulder level pulleys.

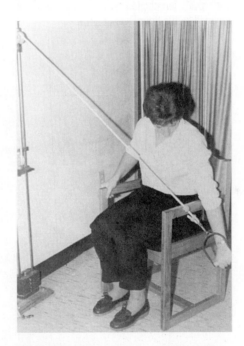

138B D1E shortened range, resistance plus a compression force.

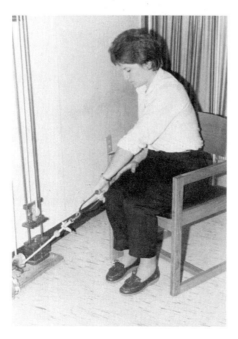

138C D2F, lengthened range, traction force provided by the floor level pulleys.

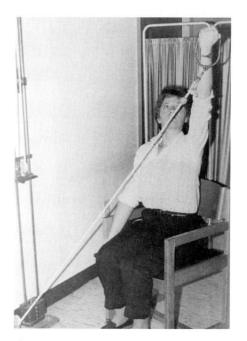

138D D2F shortened range, compression force.

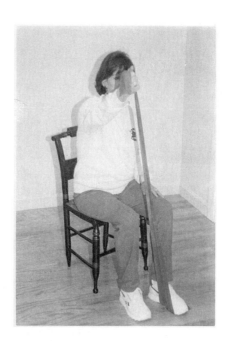

138E D2F maximum resistance midrange.

Activity: Sitting; D1 withdrawal and D1 thrust
Technique: Agonistic reversals

139

Description

The patient can be positioned in a straight-back chair or, in the case of a patient with poor sitting balance such as may occur with a patient with spinal cord injury (SCI), secured in a wheelchair. The patient is in front of the pulleys holding onto the opposite pulley handle. A traction force is provided in the lengthened range (Fig. 139A) and maximum resistance to shoulder extension occurs in the shortened range of the withdrawal pattern (Fig. 139B).

Shoulder extension is important with many SCI patients. Strengthening in this range improves the patient's ability to achieve the position of supine on elbows, an important goal of treatment. Both UEs can move in a bilateral pattern or one UE can be used to provide stabilization by holding onto the wheelchair. When performed in the second manner this static–dynamic procedure can emphasize either the dynamic limb (strengthening of the shoulder musculature) or the static limb (improving proximal stability).

All of the procedures described in sitting can be performed in supine if more stabilization is needed. The scapular abduction, shoulder flexion motion can be resisted by an elastic band (Fig. 139C).

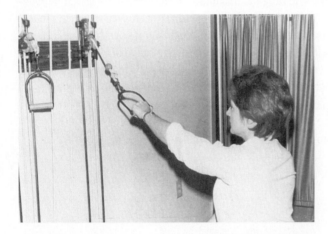

139A D1 withdrawal, lengthened range, traction force.

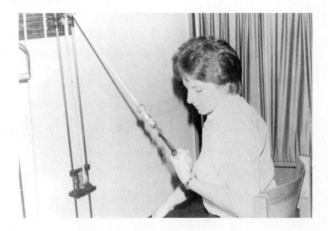

139B D1 withdrawal, shortened range.

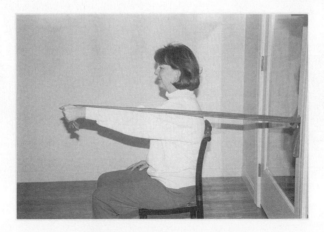

139C D1 thrust, shortened range.

Purpose/Treatment Goals

Strengthen scapular adductors, shoulder extensors, and scapular abductors and shoulder flexors, promote sitting postural control.

Lower Body Movements

140

Activity: Supine; lower trunk extension
Technique: Agonistic reversals

Description

The principles of direction of resistance and range of maximum resistance also apply to the lower extremity patterns. As with the UEs, the resistance of the pulleys is applied in a similar direction to that provided manually. Proximal resistance is provided by one overhead pulley attached to a strap around the thighs of both LEs and distal resistance is provided by the other overhead pulley line attached to foot straps.

The lower trunk extension pattern begins in the lengthened range (Fig. 140A) and moves into the shortened range (Fig. 140B). The range of maximum resistance can be varied by moving the plinth. With the pulley directly over the distal segment, maximal resistance occurs in the shortened range of the extensor pattern. If the plinth is moved so that the overhead pulleys are aligned over the hips then compression is increased in the shortened range of extension.

The angle of resistance always can be changed by moving the plinth closer to or away from the wall. An alternate method of changing the resistive angle is to combine the resistance from the overhead and shoulder level pulleys. Abduction–adduction resistance at the hip is increased by moving the plinth away from the wall and attaching the shoulder level pulley to the thigh strap. The distal resistance is still provided by the overhead pulley (Figs. 140C, 140D).

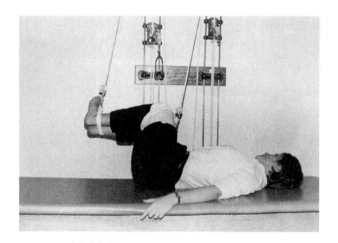

140A Lower trunk extension, lengthened range.

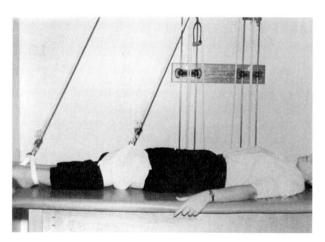

140B Lower trunk extension, shortened range.

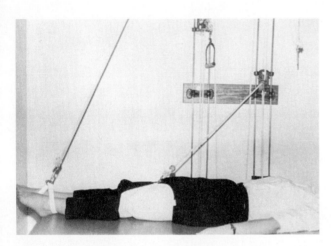

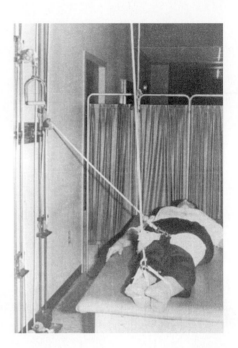

140C Resistance to extension provided by the overhead pulley and to abduction by the shoulder level pulley.

140D The resultant resistance demonstrated.

Purpose/Treatment Goals

Strengthening of the lower trunk and lower extremity extensors. If the patient is weak or if movement through range is not indicated, the hip and knee extended position can be maintained as the amount of weight is increased.

Activity: Prone; knee extension and flexion
Technique: Agonistic reversals

141

Description

In this procedure both the pulley level and the position of the patient can be changed so that knee flexion or extension can be resisted with maximum resistance occurring at different points in the range. A clinical example is the treatment plan for a patient with weak quadriceps; resistance is applied first in the shortened range of extension where inhibitory influences are minimal. As strength increases, resistance in more lengthened ranges can be added to the program.

To resist the shortened range of knee extension, the plinth is positioned perpendicular to the wall. The patient is prone facing away from the pulleys and the overhead pulley is directlly above the foot. Resistance from the overhead pulley is applied to movement from midrange to shortened range of knee extension (Fig. 141A).

To increase resistance in the midranges the patient is turned and now faces the pulley. The overhead pulley again is used. This position maximizes resistance at 45 degrees of knee extension and increases the compression force in the shortened range.

To maximally resist the quadriceps at 90 degrees of knee flexion, the patient faces toward the pulleys and the shoulder level pulleys are used (Fig. 141B). In the shortened range of knee extension a compression force is applied (Fig. 141C).

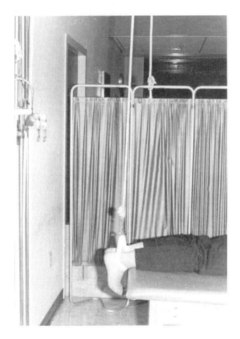

141A Knee extension, resistance maximum in shortened range overhead pulleys (the position can be maintained against increasing amounts of resistance if movement is not indicated).

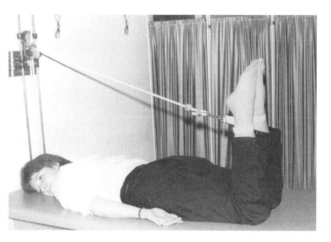

141B Knee extension, maximum resistance lengthened range, shoulder level pulleys.

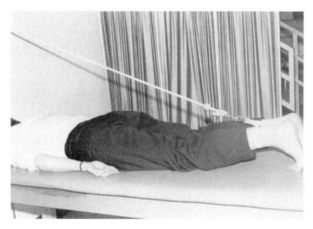

141C Resistance plus compression in the shortened range of knee extension, shoulder level pulleys.

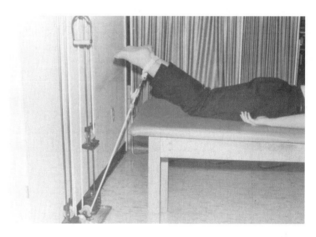

141D Midrange resistance to hamstrings, floor level pulleys.

Eccentric resistance to the hamstrings in the lengthened ranges is frequently included in treatment. To accomplish this the patient faces away from the pulleys with the feet over the edge of the plinth. Resistance is provided by the floor level pulleys (Figs. 141D, 141E).

To strengthen hamstrings in more shortened ranges, resistance is provided by the shoulder level pulleys (Fig. 141F). Because a traction force occurs with this setup in midrange (Fig. 141G), resisted movement into either knee extension or flexion can be emphasized (Fig. 141H). Resistance to the hamstrings also can be provided by an elastic band (Fig. 141I).

Purpose/Treatment Goals

Increase endurance and strength of the quadriceps and hamstrings.

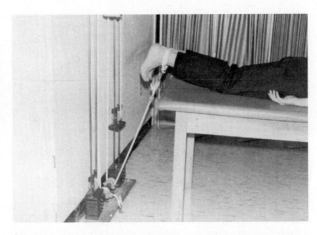

141E Lengthened range resistance to hamstrings, floor level pulleys.

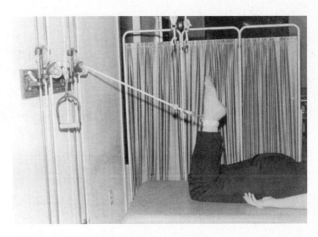

141F Shortened range resistance to hamstrings, shoulder level pulleys.

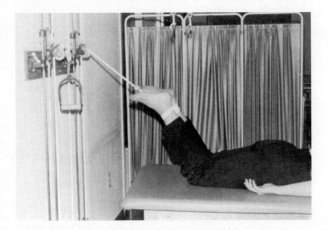

141G Midrange traction force, shoulder level pulleys.

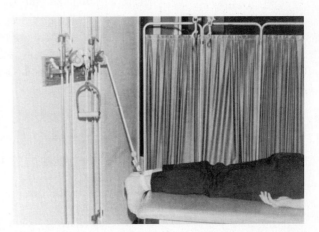

141H Shortened range resistance to quadriceps, shoulder level pulleys.

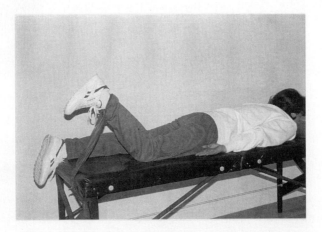

141I Lengthened to midrange resistance to hamstrings, resistive band.

142

Activity: Sitting; lower extremity extension patterns
Technique: Agonistic reversals

Description

The patient is sitting turned away from the floor pulleys with the pulley attached to the ankles. Maximal resistance occurs primarily in the midrange of knee extension with a compression force combined with resistance in the shortened range (Figs. 142A, 142B, 142C).

To emphasize resistance in the shortened range of knee extension, the plinth is pulled away from the wall and the patient faces the pulleys. The patient is positioned laterally to the pulleys so that resistance can be applied in a diagonal direction. This angled resistance may be important if facilitation of one portion of the quadriceps is desired. For example, some patients with patellofemoral arthralgia have an imbalance of strength between the vastus medialis and vastus lateralis resulting in improper tracking of the patella during active knee extension. To increase the strength of the vastus medialis the patient should be angled to promote activation of that portion of the quadriceps. If resistance through full range is not desired, a stool can be placed under the foot so that movement is limited to shortened range (Figs. 142D, 142E).

An advantage of using pulley resistance rather than free weight progressive resistance exercise (PRE) is that pulleys allow the point of maximum resistance to be altered either by changing the patient's position or the pulley level. In addition, the distraction forces that occur with free weights may be avoided with pulleys. Elastic bands may effectively resist these movements (Fig. 142F).

In addition to the extremity patterns just discussed, total body patterns of movement can be resisted to reinforce the treatment provided by the therapist.

Purpose/Treatment Goals

Increase endurance and strengthening of quadriceps.

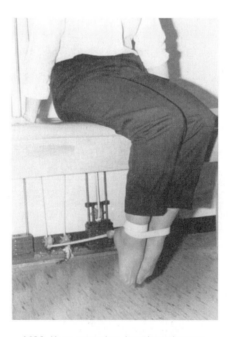

142A Knee extension, lengthened range.

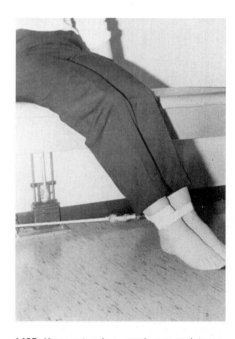

142B Knee extension, maximum resistance, midrange.

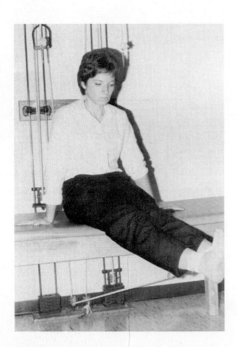

142C Knee extension, compression with resistance, shortened range.

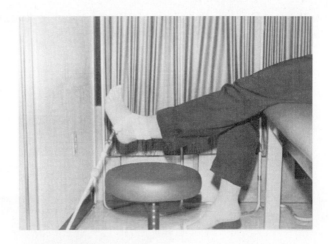

142D Unilateral knee extension, maximum resistance, mid- to shortened range.

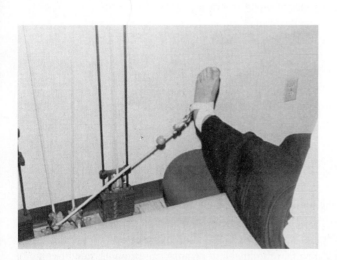

142E Angular resistance to knee extension.

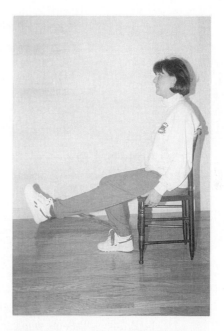

142F Knee extension, elastic band resistance.

143

Activity: Rolling; supine toward prone, D1F UE and LE
Technique: Agonistic reversals

Description

Rolling with ipsilateral D1F patterns can be resisted by attaching the foot to one floor level pulley and the hand to the other (Fig. 143A).

Purpose/Treatment Goals

Independent practice of rolling movement.

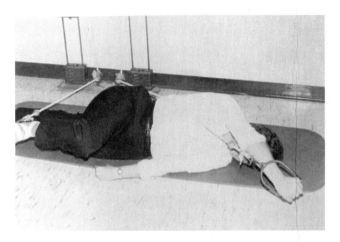

143A Rolling; supine toward prone (shortened range). The technique is AR.

144

Activity: Kneeling; assumption from heel sitting
Technique: Agonistic reversals through increments of range

Description

In this procedure the patient can practice controlled assumption and lowering from the kneeling position. The patient faces away from the pulleys. Assistance with balance and additional stabilization can be provided by holding onto a chair. Resistance at the pelvis is applied by the floor level pulleys attached to a waist strap. The resistance is similar to that applied manually in that hip and knee extensions are facilitated by an approximation or compression force (Figs. 144A, 144B, 144C). Patients who cannot maintain the kneeling posture can promote stengthening of the lower trunk and hip extensors in the bridging position (Fig. 144D).

Purpose/Treatment Goals

Strengthen hip and knee extensors in a weight-bearing position, improve independent assumption of kneeling from heelsitting.

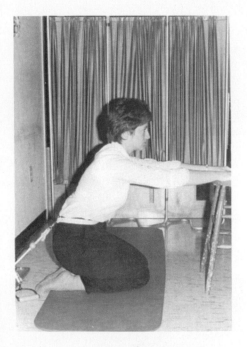

144A Heel sitting.

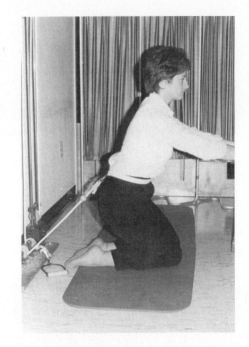

144B Midrange to kneeling.

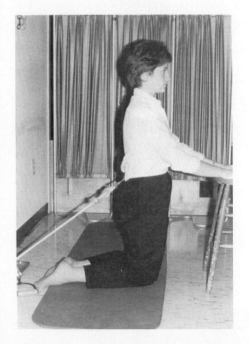

144C Kneeling.

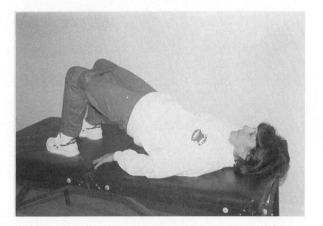

144D Bridging.

145

Activity: Prone on elbows, modified plantigrade, quadruped
Technique: Agonistic reversals to static–dynamic movements

Description

In prone on elbows the thrust/withdrawal can be resisted. In modified plentigrade upper extremity and lower extremity movements can be resisted (Figs. 145A, 145B). In quadruped, all patterns of the UEs and LEs can be resisted by altering the level of the pulley and the patient's position, or by using elastic band (Figs. 145C, 145D).

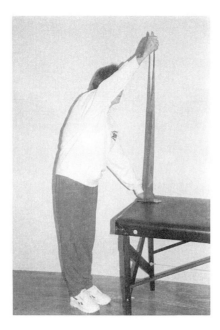

145A Modified plantigrade, unilateral D2F upper extremity.

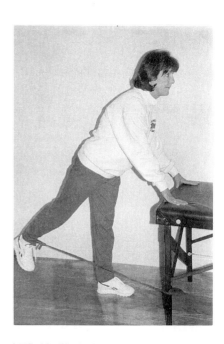

145B Modified plantigrade, unilateral D1E lower extremity.

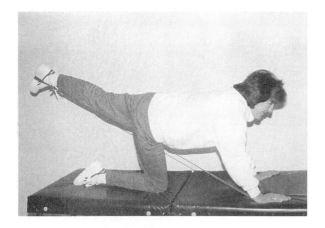

145C Quadruped; lateral limb movements.

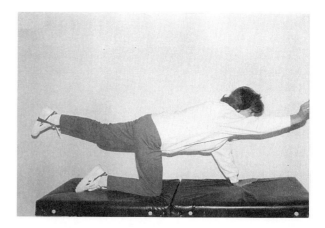

145D Quadruped; contralateral limb movements.

Purpose/Treatment Goals

Improve dynamic stability of the trunk or the static limb, or dynamic control of the moving limb.

Activity: Lower trunk rotation; lower extremity extension
Technique: Agonistic reversals

146

Description

This procedure can be used to emphasize one direction of lower trunk rotation in combination with hip abduction of one limb and adduction of the other (Fig. 146A).

Purpose/Treatment Goals

Strengthen the abdominals, the trunk and hip extensors, and one portion of the lower trunk rotation motion.

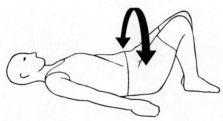

146A Lower trunk rotation; AR.

147

Activity: Standing; knee or hip flexion extension; walking in parallel bars or with walker

Technique: Agonistic reversals and resisted progression

Description

Resistance can be provided to the lower extremities while either weight bearing or moving through range. In weight bearing the challenge can be increased by the amount of band tension, by increasing the amount of weight borne through the limb or by altering the sensory input that assists postural responses (Figs. 147A, 147B, 147C).

The patient can practice resisted ambulation in the parallel bars. When the pulleys are attached to the ankles, resistance is primarily to hip flexion with knee extension. With the pulley at the pelvis, resistance to the gait pattern is combined with an approximation force (Fig. 147D).

Purpose/Treatment Goals

Improve stability around the knee, improve short arc quadriceps and hamstring control in weight bearing, increase strength of gluteus medius and gluteus maximus, challenge postural responses, enhance ambulatory ability.

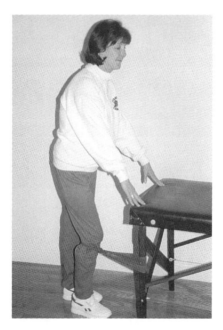

147A Band resistance to short arc knee extension.

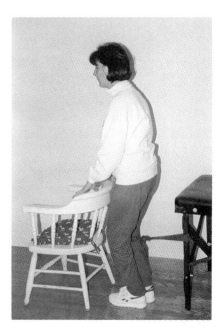

147B Band resistance to short arc knee flexion.

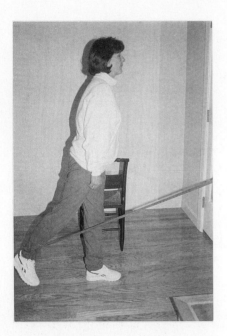

147C Band resistance to D1E.

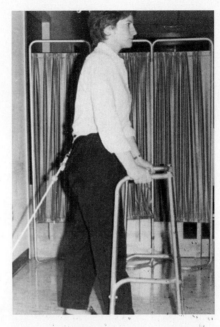

147D Pulley resistance with compression while standing.

Treatment
Sequences

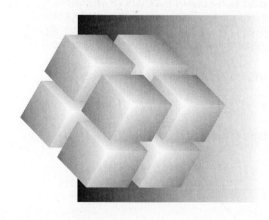

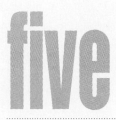

Intervention Models

Chapter Outline

INTRODUCTION

In the following section, six intervention models with examples of procedures are presented as guides to assist the therapist in deciding the treatment progression for patients with selected disabilities. The numbers in each cell of the intervention model correspond to the procedures described throughout this manual. Within the text these procedures have generally been described for a wide variety of patients. When applying each procedure the therapist must analyze and modify the treatment as needed for the particular patient's impairments to achieve the desired functional outcomes. In most situations the therapist will be overlapping many of the stages of movement control within different postures. Muscle and general body endurance may be gradually increased by altering the challenge of the movement parameters of intensity, frequency, and duration.

Shoulder Dysfunction

The intervention model for patient's with shoulder dysfunction is presented in Chart 4. The activities in this model are sequenced according to the amount of weight-bearing resistance through the limb and the amount of range of motion that occurs at the shoulder. **Mobility-ROM** is first gained in supine, sidelying, prone, or sitting with the limb nonweight bearing. Movement into flexion/adduction/external rotation, D1F, is emphasized before the more difficult and often painful movement of flexion/abduction/external rotation, D2F. In addition to the techniques to increase mobility of the musculature, the therapist may incorporate other tech-

CHART 4. Intervention Model for Patient with Shoulder Dysfunction

Activities:	Mobility		Stability		Controlled Mobility		Skill
	ROM	Initiate	Hold	Maintain	Wt. Shift	Static dynamic	
Sidelying Supine Prone Sitting	71,73 94,93	91	15 100		19 (scapular mov'ts)		70,72 78,74,75,83,86, 80,90,95 56,58,59
Sitting with upper extremity weight bearing	55		58	50	51	53	
Modified plantigrade				62	62	62	
Quadruped or standing with UE at 90 degrees against wall				31	32	34	

Parameters of Capacity — Intensity — Duration — Frequency

Stages of Control

niques, such as joint mobilization to increase the extensibility of joint and ligamentous structures. **Stability-muscle holding** is promoted in the scapular and rotator cuff musculature in non-weight-bearing postures prior to emphasizing the maintenance of weight-bearing postures. Sitting, modified plantigrade and quadruped, or standing with the arms at 90° against a wall, are a progression of postures in which the **stability, controlled mobility,** and **static–dynamic** stages of control can be sequentially promoted. **Skill** requires proximal dynamic stability. For the shoulder this ability can be described as normal scapulo-humeral rhythm. The procedures that promote skill progressively enhance control by sequencing movement from D1 to D2 and from trunk to bilateral to unilateral movement combinations.

Knee Dysfunction

The intervention model for the patient with knee dysfunction is presented in Chart 5. The activities in this model are sequenced according to the amount of weight bearing that occurs through or on the knee and the range of motion that occurs at the knee. **Mobility-ROM** is gained in the non-weight-bearing postures of supine, sitting, and prone. Joint and soft tissue mobilization can easily be included in these postures. **Stability-muscle holding** of the quadriceps and hamstrings also can be promoted in these non-weight-bearing positions. Contraction of the vastus

CHART 5. Intervention Model Knee Dysfunction

Activities:	Mobility	Stability	Controlled Mobility Wt. Shift	Static dynamic	Skill
Supine Sitting	112,121	17			109,110,111, 114,115,116, 117,118,123, 124,125
Prone	108				108
Hooklying Bridging		39,41	42,43	44	
Standing Modified plantigrade		62	62	62	65
Quadruped		31	32	34	
Kneeling		45	45	46	
Half kneeling		49	49	48	

Stages of Control

medialis oblique may be enhanced with D1F. **Stability, controlled mobility,** and **static–dynamic** stages are promoted in progressively more difficult weight-bearing, closed-chain, postures. Some patients who are elderly or who are not anticipating a return to an active lifestyle, may conclude treatment with the achievement of control in standing and modified plantigrade. Patients who need additional challenge may progress onto the postures of quadruped, kneeling, and half kneeling. Skilled movement which incorporates endurance and strength of the knee musculature can be promoted with both manually applied techniques and those that incorporate mechanical resistance including pulleys and elastic bands.

Low Back Dysfunction

The intervention model for patients with low back dysfunction is presented in Chart 6. **Mobility-ROM** of the trunk and hip musculature is promoted primarily in the non-weight-bearing postures of supine, sidelying, and prone. In these postures other treatment techniques, such as joint and soft tissue mobilization and thermal and pain-relieving modalities can be applied. **Stability-muscle holding** of the trunk extensors and abdominals are promoted in supine, sidelying, and hooklying prior to promoting isometric contractions of the extensors in the more diffi-

CHART 6. Intervention Model for Patient with Low Back Dysfunction

Parameters of Capacity — Intensity: *Gradually increasing to about 40% effort to increase endurance maintained for prolonged times to increase endurance throughout the day incorporating into functional activities* — Duration: XX — Frequency

Activities:	Mobility	Stability	Controlled Mobility	Static Dynamic	Skill
Supine Sidelying	13,105,120, 121,122	15,17,18	19		21,103,104, 106,107
Prone	26,29	23			
LTR Bridging	37	39,41	42,43	44	
Modified plantigrade		62	62	62	
Sitting		50,56,58,59	50,52	53	
Quadruped		31	32	34	
Standing		64	64		65
Kneeling Half kneel		45,49	45,46,49		

Stages of Control

cult posture of prone. **Stability, controlled mobility,** and **static dynamic** movements are promoted in progressively more difficult postures. These postures are sequenced according to many factors including the amount of weight bearing and compression that occurs through the trunk and the amount of gravitational resistance to the limb and trunk movements. Endurance of the trunk musculature is promoted as the duration, frequency, and intensity of the procedures is gradually increased.

Ankle Dysfunction

The intervention model for patients with ankle dysfunction is presented in Chart 7. Gains in **mobility** are achieved with the techniques of slow reversal (initiation of movement) and hold relax, and joint mobilization (ROM) in the non-weight-bearing postures of supine, sitting, and prone. **Stability-holding** is attained in non-weight-bearing postures to improve invertor-everter control and to enhance proprioceptive feedback. **Stability** and **controlled mobility** control are promoted in bridging, modified plantigrade, and standing. Dynamic stability, that is required during gait activities, is enhanced as maintenance and movement within these weight-bearing postures occurs. **Skill** promoted in non-weight-bearing, involves the normal distal to proximal timing of movement.

CHART 7. Intervention Model for Patients with Ankle Dysfunction

Activities:	Mobility	Stability	Controlled Mobility	Skill
Supine Sitting Prone	114,116	112		113,114,126, 127,128,129, 108
Bridging Modified plantigrade		41,62	42,44,62	
Standing		64	64	65

Parameters of Capacity — Intensity, Duration, Frequency

Stages of Control

Parkinson's Dysfunction

The intervention model for patients with impairments resulting from Parkinson's syndrome is presented in Chart 8. **Mobility** for patients with excessive tone and rigidity is promoted primarily with the technique of rhythmic initiation in non-weight-bearing postures. During the **stability** procedures the goal is to enhance holding with the postural musculature rather than with the muscles more geared toward movement. The **controlled mobility** procedures promote weight shifting and particularly trunk rotational control. **Skill** emphasizes counterrotation in the trunk and reciprocal extremity movements.

CHART 8. Intervention Model for Patients with Parkinsonism

Activities:	Mobility	Stability	Controlled Mobility	Skill
Supine Sidelying Rolling	13,22,73,72,74, 75,78,94,102,103, 107,114,118,122, 126,127,129	15,17,18	19,20	21
Prone Prone on elbows	26	23,25	27,28	
LTR Bridging	37	41	40,42,43,44	
Sitting Modified plantigrade Standing		50,58,62,64	51,52,53,54,62,64	56,59,65

Parameters of Capacity — Intensity, Duration, Frequency

Stages of Control

Hemiplegia

The intervention model for patients with hemiplegia is presented in Chart 9. Mobility for patients with abnormalities in tone is promoted primarily in postures with a large base of support and low center of gravity and incorporate techniques to promote initiation of movement out of synergistic patterns. Muscle and postural stability and controlled mobility can be promoted in progressively more difficult postures with resistance modified to prevent unwanted reactions. Skill level procedures promote functional movements, a smooth reversal of antagonists and normal timing of movement.

CHART 9. Intervention Model for Patients with Hemiplegia

Activities:	Mobility	Stability	Controlled Mobility	Skill
Supine Sidelying Rolling Prone	13,14,22,91,92,94	15,17,18,94	12,19,20,92,94	21,70,78,83,80,86, 97,98,99,102,107, 108,123,124,125, 126,127,128,129
Lower trunk rotation, bridging	37,38	39,41	40,42,43,44	
Sitting with and without UE	55,60,61	50,58	51,52,53,54,55,58	55,58,60,109,110, 111,113
Modified plantigrade		62	62	
Standing	63	64	64	65
Kneeling, Quadruped		45,31	45,46,47,48,32,35	

Parameters of Capacity — Intensity, Duration, Frequency

Stages of Control

Spinal Cord Injury

The intervention model for patients with spinal cord injury is presented in Chart 10. All levels of control are emphasized in those postures which provide the patient with optimum support. The difficulty of the procedure is largely determined by the level of the lesion. Techniques which promote overflow from stronger to weaker segments are emphasized to maximize strength and function.

CHART 10. Intervention Model for Patients with Spinal Cord Injury

Activities:	Mobility and Strengthening	Stability	Controlled Mobility	Skill
Supine, Sidelying, Rolling	13,14,22,69,72,74,75, 76,77,78,81,84,85,87, 88,89,90,94,96,97,98	15,17	19,20	21
Prone, Prone on elbows, Quadruped	24,30	25,31	27,28,32,34	
Sitting	56,57,58,59	50	51,53,54	

Parameters of Capacity — Intensity, Duration, Frequency

Stages of Control

Bibliography

Angel RW. Antagonistic muscle activity during rapid arm movements: Central versus proprioceptive influences. *J Neurol Neurosurg Psychiatry.* 1977;40:683–686.

Astrand PO, Rodahl K. *Textbook of Work Physiology.* New York, NY: McGraw-Hill Book Co; 1986.

Balance Proceedings of the APTA Forum. Alexandria, Va: American Physical Therapy Association, 1990.

Barnes MR, Crutchfield CA, Heriza CB, et al. *Reflex and Vestibular Aspects of Motor Control, Motor Development and Motor Learning.* Atlanta, Ga: Stokesville Publishing; 1990.

Bobath B. *Adult Hemiplegia: Evaluation and Treatment.* 3rd ed. London, England: Butterworth and Heinemann; 1990.

Bogduk N, Twomey LT. *Clinical Anatomy of the Lumbar Spine.* Melbourne, Australia; Churchill Livingstone; 1987.

Boissonault WG. *Examination in Physical Therapy Practice: Screening for Medical Disease.* New York, NY: Churchill Livingstone; 1991.

Brooks VB. *The Neural Basis of Motor Control.* New York, NY: Oxford University Press; 1986.

Brunnstrom S. *Movement Therapy in Hemiplegia.* New York, NY: Harper & Row Publishers Inc; 1970.

Claman PH. Motor unit recruitment and the gradation of muscle force. *Phys Ther.* 1993; 73:830–843.

Cohen M, Hoskins MT. *Cardiopulmonary Symptoms in Physical Therapy Practice.* New York, NY: Churchill Livingstone, 1988.

Crutchfield CA, Barnes MR. *The Neurophysiological Basis of Patient Treatment.* 2nd ed. Atlanta, Ga: Stokesville Publishing; 1975,1.

Cyriax JH. *Illustrated Manual of Orthopedic Medicine.* London, England: Butterworths; 1983.

Delwaide PJ, Young RR (eds). *Clinical Neurophysiology in Spasticity,* Vol. 1. New York, NY: Elsevier; 1985.

Diener HC, Dichgans JT, Guschlbauer B, et al. The significance of proprioception on postural stabilization assessed by ischemia. *Brain Res.* 1984;296:103–109.

Diener HC, Horak FB, Nashner LM. Stimulus parameters on human postural responses. *J Neurophysiol.* 1988;59:1888–1905.

Duncan P, Badke MB. *Stroke Rehabilitation: The Recovery of Motor Control.* Chicago, Ill: Year Book Medical Publishers; 1987.

Feldman RG, Young RR, Koella WP, eds. *Spasticity: Disordered Motor Control.* Chicago, Ill: Year Book Medical Publishers; 1980.

Frankel VF, Nordin MA. *Basic Biomechanics of the Skeletal System.* Philadelphia, Pa: Lea & Febiger, 1989.

Grimby L, Hannerz J. Tonic and phasic recruitment order of motor neurons in man under normal and pathological conditions. In: Desmedt JE, ed. *New Developments in Electromyography and Clinical Neurophysiology.* Basel, Switzerland: Karger; 1973.

Guccione AA. Physical therapy diagnosis and the relationship between impairments and function. *Phys Ther.* 1991; 71:499–504.

Guccione AA, ed. *Geriatric Physical Therapy.* St. Louis, Mo: CV Mosby Co; 1993.

Gordon T, Mao J. Muscle atrophy and procedures for training after spinal cord injury. *Phys Ther.* 1994;74:50–60.

Gould MJ, ed. *Orthopedic and Sports Physical Therapy.* 2nd ed. St. Louis, Mo: CV Mosby Co; 1990.

Heiniger MC, Randolph SL. *Neurophysiological Concepts in Human Behavior—The Tree of Learning.* St. Louis, Mo: CV Mosby Co; 1981.

Henneman E. Peripheral mechanisms involved in the control of muscle. In: Mountcastle VB, ed. *Medical Physiology.* 13th ed. St. Louis, Mo: CV Mosby Co; 1974;1.

Higgins S. Motor control acquisition. *Phys Ther.* 1991;71:123–139.

Hoppenfeld S. *Physical Examination of the Spine and Extremities.* 2nd ed. Norwalk, Conn: Appleton-Century-Crofts; 1976.

Horak FB. Clinical measurement of postural control in adults. *Phys Ther.* 1987;67:1881–1885.

Inman VT, Ralston HJ, Todd F. *Human Walking.* Baltimore, Md: Williams & Wilkins; 1981.

Irwin S, Tecklin JS, eds. *Cardiopulmonary Physical Therapy.* 2nd ed. St. Loius, Mo: CV Mosby Co; 1990.

Jette AM. Measuring subjective clinical outcomes. *Phys Ther.* 1989;69:580–584.

Joseph JA, ed. *Central Determinants of Age-Related Declines in Motor Function.* New York, NY: Academy of Sciences; 1988.

Kaltenborn FM, Evjenth O. *Manual Mobilization of the Extremity Joints: Examination and Basic Treatment Techniques.* Oslo, Norway: Olaf Norlis Borhandel; 1989.

Kandel ER, Schwartz JH, Jessell TM. *Principles of Neural Science.* 3rd ed. Norwalk, Conn: Appleton & Lange; 1991.

Kendall FP, McCreary EK. *Muscles: Testing and Function.* 4th ed. Baltimore, Md: Williams & Wilkins; 1993.

Kelso JAS. *Human Motor Behavior: An Introduction.* London, England: Lawrence Erlbaum Associates; 1982.

Kispert CP. Clinical measurements to assess cardiopulmonary function. *Phys Ther. 1987;67:1886–1890.*

Knott M, Voss DE. *Proprioceptive Neuromuscular Facilitation.* 2nd ed. New York, NY: Harper & Row Publishers Inc; 1968.

Langer S, Wernick J. *A Practical Manual for a Basic Approach to Biomechanics.* Wheeling, Ill: Langer Biomechanics Group; 1989.

Macefield G, Hagbarth KE, Gorman R, et al. Decline in spindle support to alpha motorneurons during sustained voluntary contractions. *J Physiol.* 1991;440:497–512.

Manual Therapy: Special Series. *Phys Ther.* 1992;72:839–967.

McComas AS, Sica REP, Upton ARM, et al. Functional changes in motoneurons of hemiparetic patients. *J Neurol Neurosurg Psychiatry.* 1973;36:183–193.

McGee JD. *Orthopedic Physical Assessment.* Philadelphia, Pa: WB Saunders Co; 1987.

Michlevitz SL. *Thermal Agents in Rehabilitation.* 2nd ed. Philadelphia, Pa: FA Davis Co; 1990.

Mohr JP. *Manual of Clinical Problems in Neurology.* 2nd ed. Boston, Mass: Little, Brown; 1989.

Mooney V. On the dose of therapeutic exercise. *Top Rehabil.* 1992;15:653–656.

Nashner LM. Strategies for organization of human posture. In: Igarashi M, Black FO, eds. *Vestibular and Visual Control on Posture and Locomotor Equilibrium.* Basel, Switzerland; S Karger Publications; 1985.

Nashner LM. Organization of human postural movements during standing and walking. In: Grillner S, Stein P, Stuart D, et al, eds. *Neurobiology of Posture and Locomotor Equilibrium.* New York: Macmillan Press; 1986.

Norkin CC, Levangie PK. *Joint Structure and Function: A Comprehensive Analysis.* 2nd ed. Philadelphia, Pa: FA Davis Co; 1992.

Portney LG, Sullivan PE. *EMG Analysis of Ipsilateral and Contralateral Shoulder and Elbow Muscles During the Performance of PNF Patterns.* Presented at the Annual Conference of the Society for Behavior Kinesiology. Boston, Mass; 1980.

Portney LG, Watkins MP. *Foundations of Clinical Research: Applications to Practice.* Norwalk, Conn: Appleton & Lange; 1993.

Proceedings of the 11-Step Conference. Alexandria, Va: Foundation for Physical Therapy; 1991.

Rothstein JM, ed. *Measurement in Physical Therapy.* New York, NY: Churchill Livingstone; 1985.

Rothstein JM, Lamb RL, Mayhew TP. Clinical uses of isokinetic measurements: critical issues. *Phys Ther.* 1987;67:1840–1844.

Schmidt RA. *Motor Control and Learning: A Behavioral Emphasis.* Champaign, Ill: Human Kinetics; 1988.

Skeletal Muscle: Special Series. *Phys Ther.* 1993;73:826–967.

Sharpe M (ed.) *The Lumbar Spine Stabilization Training and the Lumbar Motion Segment, AUS J of Physiotherapy Monograph #1*, 1995.

Smidt GL. *Gait in Rehabilitation.* New York, NY: Churchill Livingstone; 1990.

Soderberg GL. *Kinesiology: Application to Pathological Motion.* Baltimore, Md: Williams & Wilkins; 1986.

Stauber WT. Eccentric action of muscles: Physiology, injury and adaptation. In: Pandolf KB, ed. *Exercise and Sports Sciences Reviews.* Baltimore, Md: Williams & Wilkins; 1989.

Stewart DL, Abeln SH. *Documenting Functional Outcomes in Physical Therapy.* St. Louis, Mo: CV Mosby Co; 1993.

Sullivan PE, Markos PD, Minor MAD. *An Integrated Approach to Therapeutic Exercise: Theory and Clinical Application.* Reston, Va: Reston Publishing Co; 1982.

Sullivan PE, Markos PD. *Clinical Procedures in Therapeutic Exercise.* Norwalk, Conn: Appleton & Lange; 1987.

Sullivan PE, Markos PD. *Clinical Procedures in Therapeutic Exercise.* Stamford, Conn: Appleton & Lange; 1996.

Tappan FM. *Healing Massage Techniques.* 2nd ed. Norwalk, Conn: Appleton & Lange; 1988.

Thompson LV. Effects of age and training on skeletal muscle physiology and performance. *Phys Ther.* 1994;74:71–81.

Umphred DA, ed. *Neurological Rehabilitation.* St. Louis, Mo: CV Mosby Co; 1985.

Vaughan CL, Murphy GN, du Toit LL. *Biomechanics of Human Gait: An Annotated Bibliography.* Champaign, Ill: Human Kinetics; 1987.

Voss DE, Ionta MK, Myers BJ. *Proprioceptive Neuromuscular Facilitation Patterns and Techniques.* 3rd ed. New York, NY: Harper & Row Publishers Inc; 1985.

Watts NT. Clinical decision analysis. *Phys Ther.* 1989;69:569–576.

Winstein CL. Knowledge of results in motor learning: implications for physical therapy. *Phys Ther.* 1991;71:140–149.

Wolf SL. *Clinical Decision Making in Physical Therapy.* Philadelphia, Pa: FA Davis; 1985.

Wyke B. Articular neurology—a review. *Physiotherapy.* 1972;58:94–99.

The following theses by graduate students at Boston University were used as a basis for much of the material in this text. Most of this research was conducted under the supervision of Leslie Gross Portney, Patricia E. Sullivan, and Prudence D. Markos.

Batchelder ME: EMG analysis of exercise overflow in the preferred and nonpreferred leg during maximal and submaximal isometric knee extension. 1983

Barry G: EMG study of overflow during submaximal to maximal isometric knee extension. 1983

Bell TA: Trunk muscle activity and range of motion of three lumbar spinal extension exercises. 1981

Bender JM: Postural responses to self-displacement of the center of gravity tested toward the preferred and nonpreferred sides. 1982

Bernier S: Effects of contract–relax at different muscle lengths. 1980

Butterfield LS: Postural response to reaching while on a stable surface over three trials. 1982

Cotta S: Biomechanical and flexibility assessment of people with patellofemoral arthralgia. 1983

Dacko SM: Effects of force levels and rates of isometric contraction of overflow patterns in the upper extremity. 1983

Daniell JL: EMG analysis of the vastus medialis oblique and vastus lateralis in normals and subjects with chondromalacia. 1983

Dent P: EMG analysis of quadriceps activity following an isometric hold and isotonic contraction. 1980

Dirocca S: Contralateral effects of isometric contractions of the lower extremity in trained and untrained individuals. 1982

Edwards E: Postural responses of adult males and females during a lateral reaching task. 1982

Ferdiand RA: Comparison of EMG activity of the deltoid muscle during PNF and sagittal plane patterns of movement with surface and indwelling electrodes. 1979

Fine DL: Electrical activity of tonic postural muscles during prone postures. 1976

Flanagan DJ: Effects of hold–relax on straight leg raise over time. 1983

Francis NJ: EMG activity of shoulder muscles during upper extremity unilateral and bilateral PNF patterns. 1980

Herman H: EMG and torque analysis of the pubococcigeal muscle. 1982

Kluss M: Biofeedback relaxation training in subjects with bruxism. 1982

Koga KM: Timing and sequencing of exercise overflow elicited by maximal voluntary contraction. 1983

Konecky CM: EMG study of abdominals and back extensors during lower trunk rotation. 1980

Langham T: EMG analysis of hip muscles during bridging when techniques are applied. 1981

Laskas CA: Effects of a neurodevelopmental treatment on the lower extremity of a child with spastic quadriplegia. 1982

Lee CE: Effects of vibration on dynamic balance. 1984

Manske NG: Effects of a topical anesthetic on the tonic vibratory reflex in normals. 1984

Markos P: Comparison of hold–relax and contract–relax and contralateral effects. 1977

Michaels JA: Exercise overflow: An EMG investigation of a clinical procedure for indirectly eliciting contractions of the gluteus maximus and vastus medialis. 1978

Mullen SL: Neurodevelopmental treatment techniques and dorsiflexor activity in a child with spastic diplegia. 1981

Nip PS: Bilateral EMG activity of concentric, eccentric, and isometric contractions during unilateral performance of upper extremity PNF patterns. 1978

O'Connor P: Contralateral effects of isometric contractions in swimmers. 1981

Pauley LE: Monosynaptic stretch reflex and tonic vibration reflex of the biceps brachii following topical anesthesia of upper extremity skin areas. 1980

Phillips SL: EMG activity of the vastus medialis oblique relative to the vastus medialis longus, vastus lateralis, and rectus femoris during knee extension exercises. 1981

Pink M: Contralateral effects of upper extremity PNF patterns. 1978

Reich IS: Quantitative measures of force development in response to intensity of command. 1980

Rich CH: EMG study of four trunk muscles during bridging and application of alternating isometrics and rhythmic stabilization. 1981

Sargent L: EMG study of contralateral overflow during varied intensities of isometric knee flexion. 1983

Schunk MC: EMG study of the peroneus longus during bridging activities. 1981

Sever MJ: Postural responses of older adults during a lateral reaching task. 1982

Shaker JJ: EMG activity of hamstrings during knee flexion and a comparison of knee flexion to knee extensor muscle torque in normal and chondromalacia subjects. 1983

Shapiro CH: Effects of hold–relax at different muscle lengths. 1978

Shaw JA: Effect of intraday and interday applications of vibration on the tonic vibration reflex. 1980

Slavin MD: The influence of proprioceptive afferent stimulation on torque production. 1981

Smith SE: Development of extension in the prone position in infants 2–8 weeks. 1982

Taylor ON: Effects of vibration applied to physiologically different muscles. 1978

Troy L: EMG study of quadriceps and hamstrings during bridging. 1981

Tynan B: EMG analysis of isometric hold compared to isometric push contractions. 1982

Van Lontregen MA: EMG analysis of overflow in shoulder muscles during PNF patterns. 1981

Watkins MP: Cocontraction and the relationship between opposing muscles. 1974

West A: Duration of effects of contract–relax. 1983

Winston MC: Electrical activity of the tibialis anterior. 1979

Zimny N: EMG analysis of scapula musculature in different postures with varied sensory input. 1980

Index

Page numbers followed by a *c* or an *f* indicate a chart or a figure, respectively.

Page numbers followed by a *c* or an *f* indicate a chart or a figure, respectively.

Page numbers followed by a *c* or an *f* indicate a chart or a figure, respectively.

Page numbers followed by a *c* or an *f* indicate a chart or a figure, respectively.

ALSO FROM APPLETON & LANGE

Clinical Decision Making in Therapeutic Exercise
Patricia E. Sullivan, PhD, PT; Prudence D. Markos, MS, PT
1996, 313 pp., 319 illus., case, ISBN 0-8385-4045-7, A4045-9

Patient Care Skills, 3/e
Mary A. Duesterhaus Minor, MS, PT; Scott Duesterhaus Minor, PhD, PT
1995, 512 pp., 732 illus., spiral, ISBN 0-8385-7709-1, A7709-7

Correlative Neuroanatomy, 22/e
a LANGE medical book
Stephen G. Waxman, MD, PhD; Jack deGroot, MD, PhD
1995, 399 pp., 340 illus., paperback, ISBN 0-8385-1091-4, A1091-6

Essentials of Neural Science and Behavior
Eric R. Kandel; James H. Schwartz; Thomas M. Jessell
1995, 743 pp., 587 illus., case, ISBN 0-8385-2245-9, A2245-7

CURRENT Diagnosis & Treatment in Orthopedics
Harry B. Skinner, MD, PhD
1995, 645 pp., 498 illus., paperback, ISBN 0-8385-1009-4, A1009-8

Physical Agents
A Comprehensive Text for Physical Therapists
Bernadette Hecox, PT, MA; Tsega Andemicael Mehreteab, PT, MS; Joseph Weisberg, PT, PhD
1994, 473 pp., 180 illus., case, ISBN 0-8385-8040-8, A8040-6

Geriatric Physical Therapy
A Clinical Approach
Carole B. Lewis, PT, GCS, MSG, MPA, PhD; Jennifer M. Bottomley, PT, MS
1994, 635 pp., 120 illus., case, ISBN 0-8385-8875-1, A8875-5

Foundations of Clinical Research
Applications to Practice
Leslie Gross Portney, MS, PT; Mary P. Watkins, MS, PT
1993, 722 pp., illus., case, ISBN 0-8385-1065-5, A1065-0

Manual for Physical Agents, 4/e
Karen W. Hayes, PhD, PT
1993, 169 pp., illus., spiral, ISBN 0-8385-6143-8, A6143-0

Clinical Electrotherapy, 2/e
Rogert M. Nelson, PhD, PT; Dean P. Currier, PhD, PT
1991, 422 pp., 106 illus., case, ISBN 0-8385-1334-4, A1334-0

Healing Massage Techniques, 2/e
Frances M. Tappan, EdD, MA
1988, 347 pp., 188 illus., paperback, ISBN 0-8385-3655-7, A3655-6

Physical Examination of the Spine and Extremities
Stanley Hoppenfeld, MD
1976, 276 pp., 621 illus., case, ISBN 0-8385-7853-5, A7853-3

Available at your local health science bookstore or call 1-800-423-1359.

Appleton & Lange • P.O. Box 120041 • Stamford, CT • 06912-0041